Oklahoma Notes

Basic Sciences Review for Medical Licensure
Developed at
The University of Oklahoma College of Medicine

Suitable Reviews for:
United States Medical Licensing Examination
(USMLE), Step 1

Oklahoma Notes

Microbiology & Immunology

Fourth Edition

Richard M. Hyde

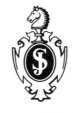

Springer-Verlag
New York Berlin Heidelberg London Paris
Tokyo Hong Kong Barcelona Budapest

Richard M. Hyde, Ph.D.
Department of Microbiology and Immunology
College of Medicine
Health Sciences Center
The University of Oklahoma
Oklahoma City, OK 73190
USA

Library of Congress Cataloging-in-Publication Data
Hyde, Richard M.
    Microbiology and immunology / Richard M. Hyde. — 4th ed.
        p.   cm. — (Oklahoma notes)
    Rev. ed. of: Microbiology and immunology. 3rd ed. c1992.
    Includes bibliographical references.
    ISBN 0-387-94392-7
    1. Medical microbiology—Outlines, syllabi, etc.   2. Medical
microbiology—Examinations, questions, etc.   3. Immunology—
Outlines, syllabi, etc.   4. Immunology—Examinations, questions,
etc.   I. Hyde, Richard M. Microbiology & immunology   II. Title.
III. Series.
    [DNLM: 1. Microbiology—examination questions.   2. Microbiology—
outlines.   3. Allergy and Immunology—examination questions.
4. Allergy and Immunology—outlines.   QW 18.2.H995m 1995]
QR46.H93   1995
616′.01—dc20
DNLM/DLC
for Library of Congress   95-2578

Printed on acid-free paper.

Production managed by Jim Harbison; manufacturing supervised by Jacqui Ashri.
Camera-ready copy prepared by the author.
Printed and bound by Edwards Brothers, Inc., Ann Arbor, MI.
Printed in the United States of America.

9 8 7 6 5 4 3 2 1

ISBN 0-387-94392-7 Springer-Verlag New York Berlin Heidelberg

Preface to the
Oklahoma Notes

In 1973, the University of Oklahoma College of Medicine instituted a requirement for passage of the Part 1 National Boards for promotion to the third year. To assist students in preparation for this examination, a two-week review of the basic sciences was added to the curriculum in 1975. Ten review texts were written by the faculty: four in anatomical sciences and one each in the other six basic sciences. Self-instructional quizzes were also developed by each discipline and administered during the review period.

The first year the course was instituted the Total Score performance on National Boards Part I increased 60 points, with the relative standing of the school changing from 56th to 9th in the nation. The performance of the class since then has remained near the national candidate mean. This improvement in our own students' performance has been documented (Hyde et al: Performance on NBME Part I examination in relation to policies regarding use of test J. Med. Educ. 60: 439–443, 1985).

A questionnaire was administered to one of the classes after they had completed the Boards; 82% rated the review books as the most beneficial part of the course. These texts were subsequently rewritten and made available for use by all students of medicine who were preparing for comprehensive examinations in the Basic Medical Sciences. Since their introduction in 1987, over 300,000 copies have been sold. Obviously these texts have proven to be of value. The main reason is that they present a *concise overview* of each discipline, emphasizing the content and concepts most appropriate to the task at hand, i.e., passage of a comprehensive examination covering the Basic Medical Sciences.

The recent changes in the licensure examination that have been made to create a Step 1/Step 2/Step 3 process have necessitated a complete revision of the Oklahoma Notes. This task was begun in the summer of 1991 and has been on-going over the past 3 years. The book you are now holding is a product of that revision. Besides bringing each book up to date, the authors have made every effort to make the tests and review questions conform to the new format of the National Board of Medical Examiners. Thus we have added numerous clinical vignettes and extended match questions. A major revision in the review of the Anatomical Sciences has also been introduced. We have distilled the previous editions' content to the details the authors believe to be of greatest importance and have combined the four texts into a single volume. In addition a book about neurosciences has been added to reflect the emphasis this interdisciplinary field is now receiving.

I hope you will find these review books valuable in your preparation for the licensure exams. Good Luck!

Richard M. Hyde, Ph.D.
Executive Editor

Preface

The material in this text has been compiled to serve as a study guide for a *review* of Microbiology and Immunology suitable for preparing for STEP 1 of the United State Medical Licensing Examination (USMLE). I have assumed that you, the reader, have already had a full fledged course covering this discipline. In-depth presentation of material will not be found in this review. You are urged to consult other study aids (lecture notes, textbooks, etc.) for detailed explanations of material that you find difficult to understand.

In general, the text of the book is on the left side of each page; questions, illustrations, summary sentences or phrases, and other study aids are on the right. This format has the intent of getting you involved in the review process. Use a highlighter, put boxes around key statements, answer the questions, and fill in the blanks as you work through the book. Your reward will be proportional to your effort (i.e., no pain, no gain). As the format is a work book, you benefit most by active participation. Write key words in the margins; add to the review statements by writing out your own; use whatever study skills you have found help you in the past.

The book is organized into three sections that reflect the balance of emphasis seen in the STEP 1 examination. Each section has a set of Review Statements at the end of the text portion; these are followed by Review Examinations which use "extended match" and "clinical vignette" formats extensively to provide the reader with practice in the test taking skills that will prove useful in the licensure examination. In addition, a comprehensive examination will be found at the end of the book. There are over 350 questions in these examinations which should provide plenty of opportunity to review and reinforce the material presented in the text. Some questions may deal with material not covered in the book; be sure that you know the answer to these questions as well, since these will expand your knowledge base further.

The section on Pathogenic Microbiology has been revised significantly. The first 18 pages are devoted to a discussion of infectious diseases by systems, starting with the Respiratory System, then progressing to Septicemia, and thence to Meningitides, much the way that pathogens invade the body. The Gastrointestinal tract is also covered, as is the Genitourinary system (with emphasis on sexually transmitted diseases). These presentations deal with the most common agents encountered, the diseases they cause, their symptoms, diagnosis, and therapy. Following these discussions the reader will find brief presentations of the major points about the individual pathogens.

Contributions by the following individuals are gratefully acknowledged: Drs. J.J. Ferretti, D.C. Graves, R.K. Tweten, and S.R. Hyde; Ms. Dawn H. Struthers (artwork); and Dr. D.R. Billington (text format). The excellent secretarial assistance of Ms. J.D. Reames is also acknowledged.

I would be sorely remiss if I did not acknowledge the enormous contributions to this text made by my wife. Her patience, understanding, and support during my hours (and days) of agony over content, illustrations, etc., were a true inspiration to me. Thanks my love!

Richard M. Hyde

Contents

Section III   Review of Pathogenic Microbiology

REVIEW OF MICROBIAL PHYSIOLOGY AND GENETICS

The first portion of this section will deal with bacteria and fungi, their structure, chemical composition, and metabolism. This will be followed by a discussion of chemotherapeutic agents that are active against bacteria, fungi and animal parasites. The second section will deal with Basic Virology (viral structure, classification, replication and the effects of antiviral agents of viral replication). The last portion will deal with Microbial Genetics (mutations, gene transfer, and recombinant DNA technologies).

BACTERIAL STRUCTURE

BACTERIAL MORPHOLOGY

Cell Wall

The cell wall of bacteria protects the cell against osmotic lysis. Both Gram positive and Gram negative bacteria have peptidoglycan (mucopeptide) as the innermost layer of the cell wall. They differ in amount, and in the nature of the surface layers.

The cell wall of Gram positive bacteria contains from 40-90% peptidoglycan, while cell walls of Gram negative bacteria contains only 5-10% peptidoglycan. In Gram positives, the next layer is carbohydrate, composed of ribitol teichoic acid, and the outermost layer of the cell wall is composed of two or three kinds of protein. The lipoteichoic acids of group A streptococcal cell walls are involved in adherence to epithelial cells.

The cell walls of Gram negative bacteria are composed of an outer layer of lipoprotein-lipopolysaccharide (endotoxin) anchored to the peptidoglycan layer (in the periplasmic space) through protein and lipoprotein molecules. The periplasmic space enables bacteria to keep various proteins close to the cell in a concentrated form (e.g. beta lactamase, etc.). The cell membrane, which is not a part of the cell wall, appears as a double layered structure immediately below the cell wall.

The basic unit of peptidoglycan is a disaccharide-tetrapeptide containing N-acetylmuramic acid, N-acetylglucosamine, D-alanine, L-alanine, D-glutamic acid or its derivative, D-isoglutamine, and a basic amino acid, usually diaminopimelic acid. The basic units of mucopeptide are cross-linked to each other to form a tight meshwork which surrounds and protects the entire cell.

Lipopolysaccharides are composed of lipid A, core and O-antigen. Lipid A is the toxic moiety of endotoxin. The polysaccharide side chains are the O antigen epitopes.

The figure below is a representation of the basic unit of peptidoglycan: NAM = N-acetyl muramic acid, NAG = N-acetyl glucosamine; the circles are the amino acids where chain cross-linking occurs, between alanine and lysine in Gram positive cocci or alanine and diamino pimelic acid (DAPA) in other bacteria.

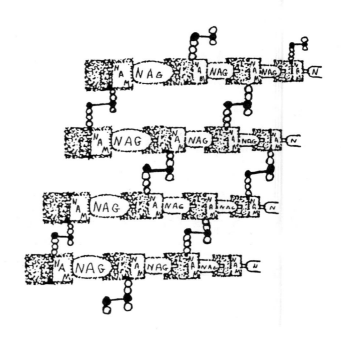

The mucopeptidase, lysozyme, hydrolyzes the linkage between N-acetylmuramic acid and N-acetyl glucosamine causing

A. the peptidoglycan layer to dissolve.
B. the cell to become osmotically-fragile.
C. Both
D. Neither

(Answer on next page)

Cytoplasmic Membrane

The ultrastructural appearance of membranes is bilayered, i.e., structures with the lipid oriented so that the non-polar (fat soluble) fatty acid side chains face the interior and the polar (water soluble) glycerol esters face the exterior of the membrane. Membrane proteins are embedded in the lipid bilayer.

Isolated cytoplasmic membranes of both Gram positive and Gram negative bacteria are approximately one-third lipid (mostly phospholipid) and two-thirds protein; occasionally polysaccharide is also attached to the membrane. There are at least three kinds of proteins associated with the cytoplasmic membranes of bacteria;
1) biosynthetic enzymes which are responsible for the synthesis of the external layers of the cell, in particular the membrane, cell wall and capsule,
2) transport proteins responsible for the transport of water-soluble materials from the medium into the cell, and
3) the cytochrome enzymes and other enzymes of the electron transport system.

The cytoplasmic membrane is a complex biologically active structure; it acts as a permeability barrier. The lipid bilayer acts as a barrier to the passage of water-soluble chemicals. A second function of the cell membrane is to serve as a site for synthesis of peptidoglycan, lipopolysaccharide and capsule. The third important function of the cell membrane is to serve as the site of electron transport and oxidative phosphorylation in aerobic and facultative bacteria.

Mesosomes

Mesosomes are invaginations of the membrane whose function is unclear. These sac-like structures are low in enzyme content. Septal mesosomes appear to be involved in cell division (they are associated with DNA).

The outer membrane of the cell wall of Gram negatives is somewhat selective, and is not as permeable to antibiotics as is the cell wall of Gram positives. Hence, the former organisms have become more important in human medicine during the antibiotic era.

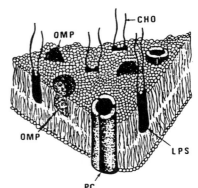

OUTER MEMBRANE OF
GRAM NEGATIVE CELL WALL

PC=PORIN PROTEIN CHANNEL
OMP=OUTER MEMBRANE PROTEIN
LPS=LIPOPOLYSACCHARIDE
CHO=CARBOHYDRATE SIDE CHAIN
OF LPS

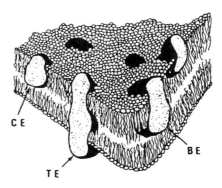

CYTOPLASMIC MEMBRANE
CE = CYTOCHROME ENZYMES
TE = TRANSPORT ENZYMES
BE = BIOSYNTHETIC ENZYMES

Answer to question about lysozyme's effect on bacterial cell wall = C.

3

INTRACYTOPLASMIC STRUCTURES

Bacterial Nucleus (Nucleoid)

The double-stranded DNA of bacteria is circular; there are usually 1-3 copies per cell. The highly coiled DNA strand is not enclosed in a nuclear membrane; DNA-associated histones are also absent. It is attached to the membrane and has associated a high mRNA content (20%).

Ribosomes

Ribosomes are the only structural organelle in the bacterial cytoplasm. They are numerous, and mostly grouped in chains (polysomes).

Cytoplasmic Inclusions

Several species of bacteria form lipid inclusions which appear to be a source of reserve energy for the organism. Metachromatic granules are composed of polymetaphosphate. The function of meta-chromatic granules is not clear, but may be related in some fashion to energy metabolism. Starch or glycogen granules have also been detected in bacteria.

Spores

Most spore-forming bacteria are Gram positive rods (Bacillus and Clostridium). They are composed of a bacterial nucleoid surrounded by a cell membrane and several layers known as the outer and inner coats which appear to be composed of highly stable proteins such as keratin, possibly with some phospholipoprotein containing Ca^{++} dipicolinate. The mature spore is a dormant organism characterized by a very low water content and metabolic rate. Spores are highly resistant to heat, light, and other deleterious agents. Spores contain the same catabolic and anabolic enzymes as do vegetative cells, but do not contain respiratory enzymes. They are formed by the parent vegetative cell in response to an adverse environmental condition such as depletion of C source.

PROKARYOTES VS EUKARYOTES

Bacteria (Prokaryotes) lack:
1. nuclear membrane
2. DNA-associated histones
3. introns in genes
4. steroids in cell membrane
5. phosphatidyl choline in membrane
6. mitochondria
7. endoplasmic reticulum

Bacteria have:
1. polygenic mRNA
2. formylmethionyl is initiator tRNA instead of methionyl
3. 70S ribosomes instead of 80S
4. Unique components of cell wall
   a. peptidoglycan
   b. diaminopimelic acid

Germination occurs in three stages.
1. Activation - caused by damage to the spore coat
2. Initiation - needs a nutritionally favorable environment. An autolysin is activated which degrades the cortex peptido-glycan. Water is taken up and calcium dipicolinate released.
3. Outgrowth - the spore protoplast emerges and active biosynthesis occurs.

EXTERNAL STRUCTURES

Flagella

Flagella, the organelles responsible for motility of bacteria, are located either at the ends of the cell (polar flagellation) or over the entire surface (peritrichous flagellation). There are three parts of the flagellum; filament, hook and basal body. The basal body arises in the membrane and is anchored in the cell wall; it is the motor.. The flagellar filament is composed of an elastic protein named flagellin; these are the H antigens of bacteria.

Axial Filaments

The organelles responsible for motility of spirochetes are called axial filaments. They are composed of protein and have a hook at the proximal end which is attached to the cell.

Pili (Fimbriae)

Pili are short, hair-like, protein structures which occur on a large number of bacterial species. Host cell selectivity may be directed by pili, e.g., the pili of the gonococcus has an affinity for the columnar epithelium of the urethra.

The sex pilus is found only on male strains of bacteria which are capable of donating their DNA by conjugation. These pili are usually named after the fertility agent carried by the strains such as F pilus and Hfr pilus. DNA of the donor is transferred to the recipient after the cells are brought into intimate contact by contraction of the sex pilus.

In streptococci, fimbriae are the site of the major surface antigen, the M protein. Lipoteichoic acid, associated with these fimbriae, is responsible for the adherence of group A streptococci to epithelial cells of their hosts.

Bacterial chemotaxis occurs when attractants (e.g. sugars) or repellents (e.g., toxic metabolites) react with chemoreceptors in the membrane or periplasmic space. Methyl-accepting proteins relay signals from the receptors to the flagellar apparatus. S-adenosyl methionine serves as the methyl donor. The signal influences flagellar rotation such that the organism moves toward, or away from, the attractant or repellent depending upon the direction of rotation of the flagella. This is an energy dependent event.

The basic mechanism of chemotaxis is hypothesized to function as follows: The chemotaxins arrive in the periplasmic space following passage through porin channels. Here they interact with periplasmic binding proteins which deliver them either to membrane transport proteins for passage into the cell or to chemoreceptor proteins of the chemotaxis system. When this occurs it exposes methylation sites on the cytoplasmic side of the receptor which are methylated by an enzyme called CheR. A series of methylation and phosphorylation events transmit the signals for directional rotation in the cytoplasm of the cell. At least five additional proteins are involved; CheY and CheZ control the direction of rotation. Phosphorylated CheY is thought to interact directly with the motor-switch complex to cause clockwise rotation. CheZ accelerates CheY dephosphorylation, thus favoring counterclockwise rotation and active "swimming" toward an attractant. The cells appear to "tumble" when the direction of flagellar rotation is reversed as would occur upon the addition of a repellant or the absence of an attractant.

Capsule

Capsules of most species of bacteria are polysaccharide, but in the genus Bacillus, there are capsules of poly D-glutamic acid. Polysaccharide capsules vary from relatively simple structures such as hyaluronic acid which is a linear polysaccharide composed of N-acetylglucosamine and glucuronic acid, to the highly branched polysaccharides formed by Streptococcus pneumoniae. Although there are usually no more than three or four sugars in capsules of S. pneumoniae, they are branched polysaccharides and are unique enough that specific antisera to the capsules can be formed. Some 80 strains of S. pneumoniae have been identified on the basis of the antigenic properties of their capsules.

Capsules of certain species of bacteria inhibit phagocytosis and thereby enhance the ability of the organism to establish an infection, i.e., they are antiphagocytic virulence factors.

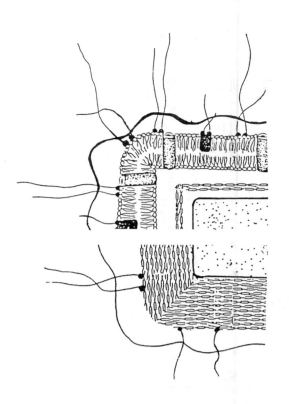

COMPARATIVE ANATOMY OF BACTERIA

Cross sections of Gram negative (top) and Gram positive (bottom) bacteria are shown in the upper right quadrant. Note the striking differences in the cell wall composition; e.g., the large amount of peptidoglycan in the Gram positive vs. the presence of the periplasmic space in the Gram negative, etc. In the diagram below the common and unique features of both groups of organisms have been listed for your edification. Label the structures in the figure in the upper right hand corner.

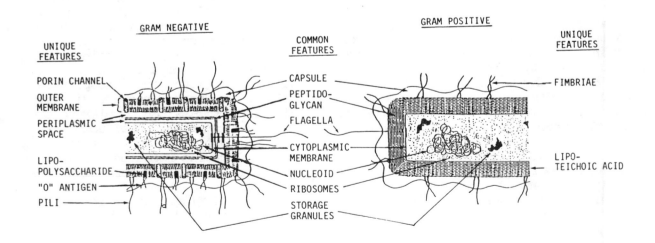

6

BACTERIAL GROWTH

GROWTH OF BACTERIA

Source of Carbon

Autotrophs are organisms which are able to use carbon dioxide as the sole carbon source. Heterotrophs require the major portion of their carbon in the form of organic carbon although almost all heterotrophs require some carbon dioxide.

Microorganisms which are pathogenic for man are heterotrophs/autotrophs?
   (Choose One)

Physical Requirements for Growth

The temperature for optimum growth of most bacteria is between 20-40 C; these are mesophiles. Bacteria which grow in association with warm blooded animals have optimum growth temperatures in the vicinity of 35-40 C.

Microorganisms which are pathogenic for man are mesophiles/psychrophiles?
   (Choose One)

The growth rate is affected by the osmotic pressure of the medium. Most bacteria are able to tolerate 1-2% salt, but the growth drops off rapidly as the salt concentration increases above this level. Haloduric organisms (e.g., S. aureus) can grow in the presence of high salt concentrations

Certain pathogenic microorganisms are haloduric; this fact is used in the design of selective media for their isolation from clinical specimens. Name a medium used for Staphylococcus aureus:

_____

The effect of pH on the growth of bacteria is as might be predicted - bacteria grow best at pH values near neutrality

Bacteria which require oxygen for growth are aerobes; strict aerobes will grow only in the presence of oxygen. Bacteria which grow in the absence of oxygen are anaerobes. Strict anaerobes are unable to grow in the presence of oxygen and are apparently poisoned by it; they lack a functional electron transport system and are unable to produce energy by oxidative phosphorylation. They utilize organic compounds as H+ donors and acceptors. obligate anaerobes also lack catalase and superoxide dismutase. The latter converts toxic superoxide radicals to H_2O_2 which is then converted to H_2O and O_2 by catalase. Peroxidase also breaks down H_2O_2. in the presence of O_2 as more energy is available for growth.

What is the genus name of a strict anaerobe which is a sporeformer?

_____

What is the genus name of a strict anaerobe which predominates in the gut?

_____

(See the Pathogenic Bacteriology
   section for answers to the above)

Measurement of Bacterial Populations

Bacteria reproduce by binary fission, an asexual process which results in two genetically identical daughter cells. Each division is a generation and it follows that each generation leads to a doubling in cell count. The growth rate is the number of generations per unit time and is obtained by dividing the number of generations by the time interval required to increase the cell count to that level. The generation time is the time required for one generation.

Phases of Growth

There are four distinct phases of growth. The first phase of growth is the lag phase. The second phase is the exponential or logarithmic phase of growth. During this phase, total and viable counts are very nearly equal. In the third phase of growth, the stationary phase, growth has stopped. Since growth is an exponential increase of protoplasm, the last generation will use as much as one half of the nutrients in the medium which means that the medium suddenly becomes unable to support growth. Usually, it is the energy source which becomes limiting, but it can also be a vitamin or amino acid which is necessary for growth. Growth may also stop because of an increase in toxic products such as acid.

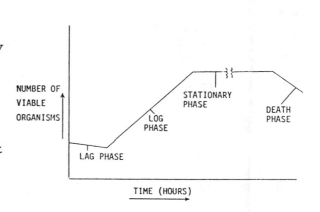

A fourth phase of the growth curve, the death phase, can occur. There is a decline in the population of bacteria. The medium is no longer able to support growth and the cell cannot maintain life indefinitely.

Sterilization and Disinfection

Sterilization involves the use of physical or chemical agents to eliminate all viable organisms; disinfection refers to the use of germicidal agents to remove the potential for infectivity of a material.

Heavy metals such as mercury are commonly used as disinfectants. Their action can be blocked by proteins or other sources of -SH groups.

Halogens such as iodine combine irreversibly with proteins and inactivate them. They also act as oxidants to destroy vital cell constituents. H_2O_2 also kills via oxidizing cellular enzymes, etc.

Alkylating agents such as formaldehyde react with proteins, nucleic acids, and other compounds with labile H+ to block their activity. These disinfectants are also blocked by proteins.

8

BACTERIAL METABOLISM

Exoenzymes

Bacteria frequently secrete enzymes which digest large, insoluble molecules into small, soluble molecules which can pass through the cell membrane.

Nutrient Transport

Kinetics - pinocytosis does not occur in bacteria and nutrients must be transported into the cell in a soluble form. Velocity of transport follows kinetics described by the Michaelis-Menten equation for enzyme reactions.

Characteristics - Bacteria use facilitated diffusion, active transport, and group translocation to transport substrates. The stereoisomer which is biologically active is selectively transported. Transport systems responsible for transport of substrates which are catabolized are usually inducible (except glucose which is constituitive.) Active transport and group translocation require energy in order to concentrate substrate inside the cell and, in the case of group translocation, to phosphorylate the substrate. Transport proteins are located in the cell membrane. Facilitated diffusion and active transport are accomplished by binding proteins which reversibly, but selectively, absorb substrate from solution.

Transport of Amino Acids occurs by active transport without chemical modification. One system may be responsible for the transport of more than one amino acid.

Transport of sugars occurs mainly by active transport and group translocation and occasionally by facilitated diffusion. Group translocation occurs only with sugars and is affected by the phosphotransferase system.

Gases (such as oxygen) water, and some ions (such as sodium) are transported into the cell by passive diffusion.

Porin channels formed by protein trimers in the outer membrane of Gram negative cell walls allow passive diffusion of molecules < 600 daltons (trisaccharides or tetrapeptides).

The four types of transport seen in bacteria are

1. _____

2. _____

3. _____

4. _____

Which of the above

- require energy?

- require a specific binding protein?

- is involved in amino acid transport?

- is involved in sodium transport?

ENERGY METABOLISM

Fermentation

Fermentation is the anaerobic metabolism
of a substrate. The Embden-Meyerhof
pathway is the most common pathway used
for sugar fermentation. Energy is
mobilized during fermentation in
phosphoryl groups of molecules such as
adenosine triphosphate and phosphenol-
pyruvate. Some anaerobic and facultative
bacteria also ferment amino acids for
energy.

Aerobic Energy Metabolism

The reduction of oxygen to water by NADH
is a rich source of energy which takes
place in aerobic and facultative bacteria
through the action of the electron
transport system. Some of the energy is
trapped by oxidative phosphorylation and
the rest is lost as heat.

The electron transport system of bacteria
is located in the cell membrane and is
composed of cytochrome enzymes, lipid
cofactors such as vitamin K and coenzyme
Q, and coupling factors, the latter being
involved in oxidative phosphorylation.

Aerobic Carbohydrate Metabolism

The most common mechanism for aerobic
metabolism of carbohydrates in bacteria
is a combination of the Embden-Meyerhof
pathway and the tricarboxylic acid cycle.
The latter is used for the aerobic
oxidation of products of the metabolism
of carbohydrates, amino acids and lipids.
Hexoses are oxidized to pyruvate, which
is oxidized to acetyl-CoA which then
enters the tricarboxylic acid cycle by
condensation with oxaloacetic acid to
citrate. Fatty acids formed by the
hydrolysis of triglycerides are also
oxidized to acetyl-CoA. Amino acids may
be oxidized to pyruvate, acetyl-CoA,
oxaloacetate, fumarate or succinate.

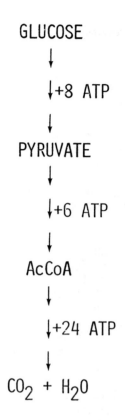

GLUCOSE
↓
↓+8 ATP
↓
PYRUVATE
↓
↓+6 ATP
↓
AcCoA
↓
↓+24 ATP
↓
CO_2 + H_2O

Which type of metabolism produces more
energy: aerobic or anaerobic?

How much more?

10

CHEMOTHERAPEUTIC AGENTS

CHEMOTHERAPEUTIC AGENTS—ANTIMETABOLITES

Sulfonamides

Action

Sulfonamides are bacteristatic, that is, they inhibit growth but do not kill; these drugs depend on the immune system of the host to remove and kill the infecting bacteria. Para-aminobenzoic acid and many other natural products such as thymine, purines, serine and methionine may overcome the action of sulfa drugs, thus sulfonamides are often found to be ineffective in sites of extensive tissue destruction. Sulfonamides inhibit the condensation of 2-amino-4-hydroxy-6-dihydropteridinyl-pyrophosphate with para-aminobenzoic acid. Sulfonamide condenses with pteridine pyrophosphate forming an analogue of dihydropteroic acid. They act as allosteric inhibitors of dihydropteroate synthetase. The drug is most effective against those bacteria which are able to synthesize their own folic acid.

The low toxicity of sulfonamides for man is understandable since man is unable to synthesize folic acid. The concentration of folic acid in tissue is either too low to reverse the action of sulfonamides or sulfa sensitive bacteria are impermeable to folic acid.

Resistance

The most frequently observed naturally occurring resistance to sulfonamides is associated with the presence of an R factor. Resistance appears to be due to the production of an altered dihydropteroate synthetase.

Clinical Use

Sulfonamides are used for urinary tract infections, some upper respiratory tract infections, for shigellosis, and for trachoma and inclusion conjunctivitis. They are also used in combination with a dihydrofolate reductase inhibitor, trimethoprim, which gives enhancement of antibacterial action.

Drugs that inhibit microbial growth but do not kill the organism are

_____.

Sulfonamide drugs are not toxic to humans because we do not synthesize

_____.

Compounds that compete with sulfa drugs and may reverse their bacteristatic action include:

1. _____

2. _____

3. _____

4. _____

5. _____

11

Other Antimetabolites

Para-aminosalicylic acid is also an analogue of para-aminobenzoic acid with many actions similar to sulfonamide. Para-aminosalicylic acid is bacteristatic and inhibits the condensation of 2-amino-4-hydroxy-6-dihydropteridinyl-pyrophosphate and para-aminobenzoic acid. The action of para-aminosalicylic is also reversed by para-aminobenzoic acid. The most important use of para-aminosalicylic acid is for the treatment of tuberculosis.

Isoniazid (INH) is a bactericidal agent which is also used for treatment of tuberculosis, frequently in combination with para-aminosalicylic acid. The mode of action of isoniazid is to inhibit synthesis of mycolic acids, an important component of the mycobacterial cell wall. INH toxicity is manifest as peripheral neuritis; it also has nephrotoxicity.

Sulfone derivatives such as diaminodiphenylsulfone (Dapsone) have been the drugs of choice for treatment of leprosy; however, recently rifampin has been used with promising results. These drugs also act as PABA antagonists.

Trimethoprim is a competitive inhibitor of microbial dihydrofolate reductase; it has little activity against the mammalian enzyme. When combined with sulfonamides the sequential blockade of the pathway to tetrahydrofolate makes for effective synergy. Trimethoprim has broad spectrum activity, including Plasmodia and Pneumocystis carinii; it is widely used for enteric and urinary tract infections.

Which antimetabolite(s)
- inhibit dihydrofolate reductase?

- inhibit dihydropteroic acid synthetase?

- inhibit mycolic acid synthesis?

--In the flow chart below--
Insert the antimetabolites on the numbered lines and the enzymes in the margins at the steps of their activity.

2-amino-4-hydroxy-6-dihydropteridinyl-pyrophosphate

+

Glutamic acid

+

Para-aminobenzoic acid

1. _____

2. _____

3. _____
          ↓
   Dihydrofolic acid

4. _____
          ↓
   Tetrahydrofolic acid

CHEMOTHERAPEUTIC AGENTS - ANTIBIOTICS

INHIBITORS OF CELL WALL SYNTHESIS

Penicillins and Cephalosporins
Structure

These antibiotics have a similar chemical structure, the common élement being a beta lactam ring. They also have a similar mode of action. Benzylpenicillin, or penicillin G, has the disadvantages that it is hydrolyzed by acid, which limits its oral use, and is inactivated by penicillinase. Semisynthetic penicillins have substituted acyl groups which make them stable to acid, resistant to penicillinase, or both.

Mode of action

These are bactericidal agents which inhibit peptidoglycan synthesis. Their molecular configuration is similar to that of the D-alanyl-D-alanine terminus of the pentapeptide side chain and they react with the transpeptidase forming an inactive complex.

Resistance

Bacterial resistance to penicillins is usually the result of a lactamase whose production is governed by plasmids. Beta lactamases hydrolyze the B-lactam ring. Penicillinases are active against penicillins but relatively inactive against cephalosporins.

Clinical Use

Benzylpenicillin is used for infections caused by penicillin-sensitive organisms such as streptococci, Neisseria, and Treponema. Methicillin, oxacillin and nafcillin are used for infections caused by bacteria which form penicillinases Oxacillin has the advantage that it can be used orally. Ampicillin and Carbenicillin are more effective against Gram negative bacteria than are the other penicillins. The cepholosporins are used mostly against penicillin-resistant organisms since some penicillinases do not inactivate second and third generation cepholosporins. Cephalosporins can also be used in some allergic patients although cross reactivity does occur.

beta lactam ring

R-CO-NH—[...]—S—CH₃/CH₃ ... O=, N, COOH

R = Side chains which are added to the 6-aminopenicillanic acid core in the semisynthetic penicillins; differences here determine degree of activity, spectrum, resistance to enzymatic cleavage, and other pharmacological properties.

Clavulanic acid is a β lactam compound without significant antimicrobic activity which can bind irreversibly to the enzyme and inactive it. When given at the same time as the antibiotic, this drug protects the penicillin from enzymatic degradation.

Allergy to the penicillin antibiotics is against the 6-aminopenicillanic acid portion of the molecule or, more commonly, to its degradation products.

Resistance to penicillin is usually due an enzyme, _____ the production of which is governed by independently replicating genetic unit known as a _____ .

13

Other Inhibitors of Wall Formation

D-Cycloserine owes its antibacterial action to the fact that it is an analogue of D-alanine and competes with it for transport by the D-alanine-glycine transport system. D-Cycloserine is a competitive inhibitor of the alanine racemase and D-alanyl-D-alanine synthetase, both of which are important enzymes in the synthesis of peptidoglycan. The most important use of cycloserine is as a second line drug in the treatment of tuberculosis.

Vancomycin is an antibiotic which inhibits the transfer of the disaccharide-pentapeptide from the phospholipid carrier to the cell wall acceptor. It binds to D-alanyl-D-alanine. Vancomycin is more active against Gram positive bacteria than Gram negative bacteria.

Bacitracin is a polypeptide antibiotic produced by Bacillus species which is active against Gram positive bacteria and Neïsseria. Bacitracin is used only topically. Bacitracin inhibits the hydrolysis of lipid pyrophosphate to lipid phosphate thereby preventing its reuse in mucopeptide synthesis. It inhibits production of monophosphate carrier protein.

D-cycloserine is a competitive inhibitor of two enzymes, _____, and _____, both of which are important in _____ _____ synthesis.

Vancomycin inhibits the transfer of disaccharide-pentapeptide from the _____ carrier to the _____ acceptor.

ANTIBIOTICS WHICH INHIBIT PEPTIDOGLYCAN SYNTHESIS (BACTERICIDAL ACTION)

CYTOPLASM	MEMBRANE	CELL WALL

D cycloserine
  a competitive inhibitor
  of alanine racemase and
  D-alanyl-D-alanine
  synthetase.
	Bacitracin
	  inhibits the lysis of
	  lipid pyrophosphate
	  thereby limiting avail-
	  able substrate for muco-
	  peptide synthesis.
		Penicillins and Cephalosporins
		  react with transpeptidase
		  forming an inactive complex
		Vancomycin
		  inhibits transfer of di-
		  saccharide-pentapeptide
		  to the cell wall.

14

CELL MEMBRANE INHIBITORS

These antibiotics interact with the membrane of the cell and alter its osmotic properties. The membrane becomes "leaky" and allows the escape of K+ ions and vital metabolites, e.g. glucose. Some are also able to react with mammalian cell membranes, and hence are quite toxic.

Polymyxins are a family of decapeptides. They are active against Gram negative bacteria only. Because of the extreme toxicity, they are used primarily in the treatment of antibiotic resistant Pseudomonas infections.

Polyenes are macrolide antibiotics. The two most important are nystatin and amphotericin B. These agents selectively inhibit organisms that have ergosterol in their membranes hence they are active against the FUNGI but have no toxicity for prokaryotic forms such as bacteria due to the absence of sterols in the bacterial cell membrane. They disrupt the integrity of the sterol-containing cell membrane.
Nystatin is highly toxic and is only used for topical fungal infections (e.g., candidiasis). Amphotericin B is used parenterally; nephrotoxicity is a major complication of its use.

Imidazoles are synthetic agents which exhibit anti-fungal activity. Miconazole and ketoconazole are clinically the most useful. The former is used topically or intravenously; ketoconazole is effective when administered orally. Both of these compounds interfere with ergosterol synthesis.

Microbial and mammalian membranes are quite similar, hence drugs which affect their antibacterial action via membrane action are likely to be toxic. They cause _____ _____.

Polymyxin B is used in the treatment of infections caused by _____. Amphotericin B reacts with fungal membranes due to their content of

_____.

Ketoconazole interferes with the synthesis of _____.

REVIEW

Penicillin and other inhibitors of cell wall formation are bactericidal/bacteristatic?

Antifungal antibiotics include _____, _____, and _____.

Antifungal imidazole compounds include _____, and _____, both of which interfere with the synthesis of _____.

INHIBITORS OF PROTEIN SYNTHESIS

Streptomycin

Structure
Streptomycin is an aminoglycoside
antibiotic.

Action
Streptomycin is a bactericidal drug with
several effects on growing bacteria. The
lethal effect seems to be a result of its
inhibition of protein synthesis by preventing initiation. Streptomycin binds
to the 30S ribosome; the binding site has
been identified as a ribosomal protein
designated S12. Chromosomal mutations
may alter this binding site, producing
streptomycin resistant forms.

Resistance
One mode of resistance is an altered S12
ribosomal protein that no longer binds
streptomycin. Resistance is also associated with the presence of R factors
(plasmids) which carry genes for enzymes
that cause a chemical modification of
streptomycin making it ineffective as an
antibiotic, i.e. streptomycin-
spectinomycin adenyl transferase, streptomycin phosphotransferase and acetyl
transferase.

Clinical use
Streptomycin is bactericidal
for most Gram negative bacilli but not
for most Gram positive bacteria. It is a
first line drug for the treatment of
tuberculosis, usually with ethambutol,
rifampin, para-aminosalicylic acid and
isoniazid. Streptomycin is also used
frequently in the treatment of
genitourinary tract infections caused by
Gram negative bacilli. Streptomycin is
the drug of choice for tularemia and plague
and is used for brucellosis in combination with one of the tetracyclines.
Streptomycin,when used for long periods
of time, will cause damage to the eighth
cranial nerve, resulting in hearing loss.

Aminoglycoside antibiotics bind to the

_____ ribosome, reacting with a

ribosomal protein designated _____.

They inhibit protein synthesis by _____

_____.

Resistance to streptomycin is most

often due to enzymes produced by the

organism, namely _____,

or _____.

Streptomycin is most commonly used vs

Gram _____.

It is not effective on these bacteria

if they are growing anaerobically

(drug transport into cell requires

aerobic growth).

Aminoglycoside antibiotics are

bactericidal/bacteriostatic?

16

OTHER AMINOGLYCOSIDES

Kanamycin, Amikacin, and Gentamicin

Activity
These are also bactericidal antibiotics with an action similar to streptomycin. They also cause misreading in protein synthesis.

Resistance
Resistance to these antibiotics is associated with the presence of an R factor and is a result of the production of antibiotic modifying enzymes.

Clinical use
These antibiotics have pharmacological properties similar to streptomycin. They are bactericidal for Gram negative bacilli, mycobacteria and staphylococci.

Amikacin is used in treatment of Proteus and Pseudomonas infections. It is highly resistant to enzymatic inactivation. Gentamicin has a similar spectrum but is more readily inactivated by microbial enzymes.

The aminoglycosides are not absorbed from the intestine, hence treatment of systemic disease requires injection. They are commonly used in conjunction with B-lactam antibiotics for severe infections such as Gram negative sepsis. The basis for this synergy is the cell wall damage done by the lactam-active antibiotic facilitates aminoglycoside uptake by the offending pathogen.

Resistance to the aminoglycoside antibiotics is usually associated with a plasmid called an _____ factor. It is the result of enzymes which inactivate the antibiotic by enzymatic modifications such as

_____ ,

_____ ,

and _____ .

[see table on antibiotic resistance mechanisms at end of this section]

Aminoglycoside antibiotics have toxicity for the _____ cranial nerve, causing _____ .

Spectinomycin, although not an aminoglycoside, has some structural similarities. However, its action is bacteriostatic. It does not inhibit initiation, but does cause the formation of unstable initiation complexes. Spectinomycin is used in the treatment of gonorrhea to by-pass the problems of PPNG (see Pathogenic Bacteriology section for the meaning of this abbreviation).

TETRACYCLINES

Structure
The tetracyclines are a family of anti-biotics with a four ring structure.

Activity
Tetracyclines are active against a wide variety of microorganisms. Sensitive organisms include not only Gram positive and Gram negative bacteria, but also rickettsia, mycoplasma and chlamydia. Tetracyclines are bacteristatic drugs which inhibit protein synthesis. They bind to the 30S ribosome and inhibit binding of aminoacyl-tRNA to the acceptor site of this ribosome.

Tetracycline antibiotics bind to the 30S ribosome and inhibit binding of

_____ .

Tetracyclines are bactericidal/static?

Resistance
Resistance is associated with the presence of an R factor in Gram negative bacilli which confers resistance against all tetracyclines. Unlike other R factor-mediated resistance, however, resistance to tetracyclines appears to be due to an impaired ability to transport the drug into the cell through the cytoplasmic membrane.

Bacterial resistance to tetracyclines

is due to _____

_____ .

Clinical use
Tetracyclines are absorbed from the gastrointestinal tract, and therefore can be used orally. They are first line drugs for treatment of infections caused by rickettsia, mycoplasma and chlamydia. Tetracyclines are also used for the treatment of cholera and brucellosis and for treatment of infections caused by bacteria which have become resistant to other antibiotics.

Tetracycline drugs are active against

many bacteria, including _____ ,

_____ , _____ ,

_____ , and _____ .

A PRECAUTION ABOUT THE USE OF ANTIBIOTICS

One of the serious side effects of therapy with the tetracyclines and to a lesser extent with penicillin and the aminoglycosides is superinfection by resistant organisms. Superinfection occurs in the gastrointestinal tract, oral cavity, and vagina, usually after oral administration of antibiotics. Resistant organisms which predominate in these cases are Staphylococcus aureus, Candida albicans, Pseudomonas and Proteus. Tetracyclines are also deposited in teeth during calcification and may produce a yellow stain when used in large doses in children.

18

REVIEW OF ANTIBIOTICS WHICH AFFECT CELL WALL SYNTHESIS

Fill in the blanks with the appropriate antibiotics. (Answers on next page)

A. _____   B. _____

C. _____   D. _____

                                    UDP-N-acGlc
                                        ↓
                                    UDP-N-acMur

L-ala   ↓
                                    UDP-N-acMur-tripeptide   CYTOPLASM
  ╪   A. _____   ↓
                                    UDP-N-acMur-pentapeptide
D-ala   D-alanyl-D-ala   ↓

                                        ↓
                            Lipid-P-P-N-acMur-pentapeptide
                                        ↓
                            Lipid-P-P-N-acMur-pentapeptide-N-acGlu

        B. _____   ╪
                                    Murein   MEMBRANE

                            Lipid-P-P
        C._____   ╪

                            Lipid-P

                            Murein-pentapeptide

        D._____   ╪

                            Cross-linked Murein   CELL WALL

CHLORAMPHENICOL

Activity

Chloramphenicol is a broad spectrum antibiotic which is bacteristatic for both Gram positive and Gram negative bacteria, rickettsia and chlamydia. Chloramphenicol is one of several antibiotics which bind to the 50S ribosome, others being the macrolide antibiotics such as erythromycin and the lincomycins.. Chloramphenicol's effect on protein synthesis appears to be the result of the interference with peptide bond formation; it inhibits peptidyl transferase of the 50S Ribosome.

Resistance

Resistance to chloramphenicol in Gram negative bacilli is also associated with the presence of an R factor which is responsible for the formation of an enzyme, chloramphenicol acetyl transferase, which catalyzes the formation of the mono- and diacetyl derivatives of chloramphenicol with acetyl coenzyme A resulting in inactivation of the drug.

Clinical use

It should be used primarily for typhoid fever, H. influenzae, meningitis, anaerobic infections and for those bacterial infections resistant to other drugs. Aplastic anemia associated with the use of chloramphenicol has restricted the use of this drug.

Clindamycin, although chemically unlike chloramphenicol, has a similar mechanism of action, i.e. it inhibits peptidyl transferase of the 50S ribosome and blocks petide bond formation. The major use for clindamycin is in therapy of infections caused by anaerobes.

REVIEW OF ANTIBIOTICS THAT INTERFERE WITH PROTEIN SYNTHESIS

In the blank write the name of the appropriate antibiotic.
(answers on next page)

A. _____

B. _____

C. _____

D. _____

ANSWERS TO CELL WALL QUESTIONS
A=cycloserine
B=vancomycin
C=bacitracin
D=penicillin or cephalosporin

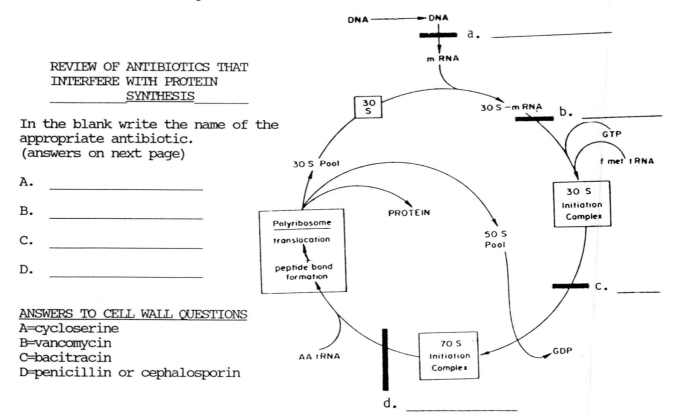

ERYTHROMYCIN

Structure
This is the most important of the macro-lide antibiotics. These agents contain a macrocyclic lactone ring to which 1 or more sugars are attached.

Activity
Erythromycin reacts with the 50S ribosomal subunit and seems to block the trans-location step in protein synthesis by inhibiting the release of charged tRNA from the donor site.

Resistance
May be either mutational or plasmid mediated. The chromosomal change which imparts resistance is due to a conforma-tional change in one of the ribosomal proteins resulting in a decrease in drug binding. Plasmid-mediated resistance is due to methylation of an adenine residue in the 23S subunit, which reduces its affinity for the antibiotic. The modified ribosomes are cross-resistant to lincomycin and clindamycin, suggesting that these two non-macrolide antibiotics have a similar site of action to that of erythromycin.

Clinical use
This bacteristatic antibiotic is used as the primary drug for M. pneumoniae infec-tions and for Legionella as well. It is also used against streptococci in patients allergic to penicillin.

GRISEOFULVIN

This is a fungistatic agent which is active against mycotic agents. It is used primarily in the treatment of dermatophyte infections. Treatment must be for a period of time (usually months) sufficient for skin or other infected tissue to be sloughed. Griseofulvin inhibits the assembly of proteins, thus it inhibits cell division by blocking the assembly of microtubules which are essential for chromosome movement during mitosis. It concentrates in keratinized layers of skin.

Chloramphenicol = bactericidal/static.

Erythromycin = bactericidal/static.

Fusidic acid is a steroid produced by the mold Fusarium. It binds to elongation factor G and blocks the growth of the peptide chain. It is used against Gram positive cocci especially penicillin-resistant Staphylococcus aureus.
[Where would Fusidic acid go in the table of page 23?]

Most antibiotics are bactericidal. Those that are not include clindamycin, chlor-amphenicol, tetra-cyclines, the sulfas and erythromycin.

Answers to protein synthesis antibiotics questions

A=rifamycin
B=tetracycline
C=aminoglycosides
D=chloramphenicol

INTERFERENCE WITH RNA SYNTHESIS

Rifampin

Activity

Rifampins are bactericidal for many species of Gram positive bacteria, Gram negative bacteria and Mycobacterium tuberculosis. Rifampins cause RNA synthesis to decrease. They inhibit the action of DNA-dependent RNA polymerase by binding to the polymerase which makes the enzyme inactive. They inhibit initiation of RNA synthesis.

Resistance

Resistance to rifampins is due to an altered B-subunit of RNA polymerase with a decreased ability to bind rifampin.

Clinical use

Rifampin is the most widely used of the rifamycins since, unlike the other rifamycins, it is readily absorbed from the intestinal tract. Its principal use is in the treatment of tuberculosis.

Antibiotics which interfere with protein synthesis include:

1. _____

2. _____

3. _____

4. _____

The major bacteristatic antibiotics include:

1. _____

2. _____

3. _____

REVIEW OF PLASMID (R FACTOR) MEDIATED ANTIBIOTIC RESISTANCE

Group	Antibiotic	Mechanism of Resistance[*]
1.	Erythromycin Clindamycin	Methylation of ribosomal RNA keeps antibiotic from binding to ribosome
2.	Sulfonamides Tetracycline	Alteration of cell membrane decreases permeability to the antibiotic
3.	Chloramphenicol	Acetylation of the antibiotic inactivates it
4.	B-Lactams	B-lactamase hydrolysis breaks down antibiotic to an inactive form
5.	Aminoglycosides	Modifying enzymes cause a) acetylation b) adenylation c) phosphorylation

[*] In addition chromosomal mutations decrease susceptibility to erythromycin, streptomycin and rifampin by altering host cell proteins to decrease drug binding. Methicillin resistance is due to a change in a penicillin-binding protein (e.g. a transpeptidase) in the cell membrane.

Antibiotic Actions

Antibiotic	Synthetic Step Blocked	Level of Blockade

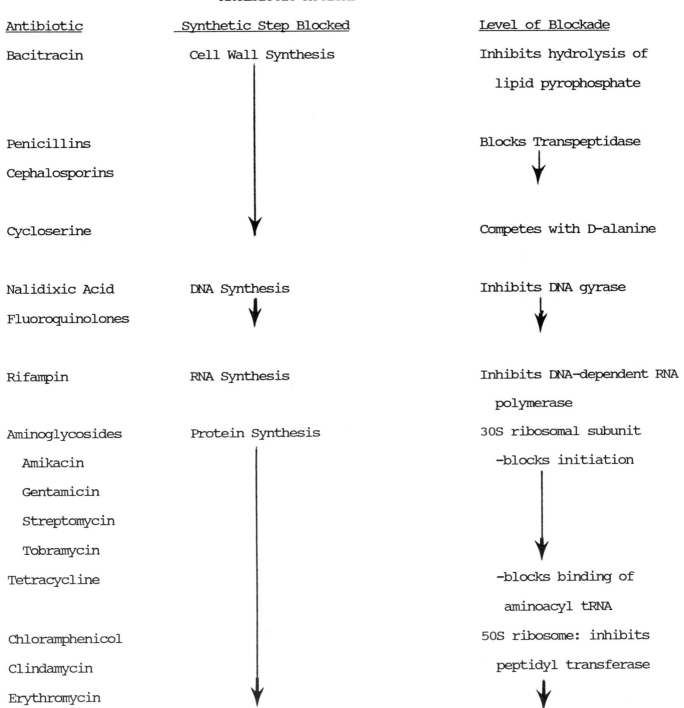

Antibiotic	Synthetic Step Blocked	Level of Blockade
Bacitracin	Cell Wall Synthesis	Inhibits hydrolysis of lipid pyrophosphate
Penicillins Cephalosporins		Blocks Transpeptidase
Cycloserine		Competes with D-alanine
Nalidixic Acid Fluoroquinolones	DNA Synthesis	Inhibits DNA gyrase
Rifampin	RNA Synthesis	Inhibits DNA-dependent RNA polymerase
Aminoglycosides Amikacin Gentamicin Streptomycin Tobramycin	Protein Synthesis	30S ribosomal subunit -blocks initiation
Tetracycline		-blocks binding of aminoacyl tRNA
Chloramphenicol Clindamycin Erythromycin		50S ribosome: inhibits peptidyl transferase

VIRAL STRUCTURE

The outermost component of a virion is the capsid, made up of protein subunits called capsomers. The capsid serves four important functions: (1) it protects the viral genome, (2) it aids in infection by attaching the virion to susceptible cells, (3) it is the stimulus for antibody production, (4) it serves as the antigen in serologic tests and (5) it is responsible for tissue tropism in naked viruses such as polio.

The viral genome, the other major component of every virion, is found inside the virus particle and may be either double-stranded or single stranded DNA, or single-stranded or double-stranded RNA. Once introduced into a susceptible cell, the viral genome provides the genetic information needed for production of new virions in a cell. The cell contributes cellular structures (ribosomes), energy, and enzymes for the synthesis of viral macromolecules. Since viruses lack most of these essential components, they must invade and make use of living cells in order to be replicated.

Animal virions are either naked or enveloped. A naked virion consists of nucleic acid enclosed in a protein shell known as the capsid; nucleic acid and capsid together are termed nucleocapsid. An enveloped virion in turn consists of a nucleocapsid surrounded by a structure called the envelope. The envelope consists of viral protein components (usually glycoproteins), and host cell-derived lipids and lipoproteins. Lipid solvents (e.g., ether) and detergents solubilize the envelope and inactivate the virus. The capsid and the envelope contribute antigens useful in vaccine development and in serologic tests.

label the components of the virus.

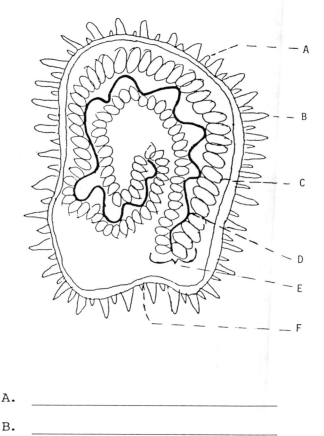

A. _____

B. _____

C. _____

D. _____

E. _____

F. _____

24

VIRAL CLASSIFICATION

All naked animal virus particles resemble icosahedra. Enveloped animal virions exhibit a large variety of shapes (symmetry). In many cases, a nucleocapsid that is distinctly icosahedral or helical, depending on the virus, is surrounded by an envelope which gives the particle the appearance of a sphere, e.g., influenza virus. Other enveloped animal viruses are shaped like a bullet, e.g., rabies virus; and still others look like bricks, e.g., poxviruses.

Taxonomic classification of viruses is based on the relatively constant physical and chemical properties of virions. Some of the criteria used for classification are (1) type of nucleic acid found in the virion (DNA or RNA) and whether the nucleic acid is single-stranded or double-stranded, (2) shape of the viral nucleocapsid (icosahedral or helical), (3) nature of the outermost viral component (naked or enveloped), and (4) antigenic properties.

Viruses are classified on the basis of

1. _____

2. _____

3. _____

4. _____

MAJOR HUMAN VIRUS GROUPS

DNA viruses

1. Herpes

    a. simplex I & II

    b. varicella

    c. cytomegalo

    d. Epstein-Barr

2. Hepadna (Hepatitis B)

3. Adeno

4. Pox

5. Papova

6. Parvo

The viral capsid has four functions:

1. _____

2. _____

3. _____

4. _____

Many viruses (e.g., the Herpes group, are inactivated by detergents and ether. This is because their outer membrane is rich in _____ .

25

RNA viruses

1. Picorna

   a. Entero
      1. Polio
      2. Coxsackie
      3. ECHO
      4. Hepatitis A
   b. Rhino

2. Toga
   a. WEE, EEE, VEE
   b. Rubella

3. Flavi
   a. Dengue
   b. Yellow fever
   c. St. Louis

4. Arena (LCM)

5. Bunya

6. Rhabdo

7. Orthomyxo

8. Paramyxo
   a. Parainfluenza
   b. Mumps
   c. Measles
   d. Respiratory syncytial

9. REO
   a. Reo
   b. Rota
   c. Orbi

10. Corona

11. Retro
    a. Oncorna (HTLV-1)
    b. Lenti (HIV)

Uncertain NA type
   1. Slow Viruses
   2. Prions (protein only)
   3. non A/non B Hepatitis
      [Hepatitis C is RNA;
      may be a Flavivirus]

The Enteroviruses are so called because they grow in the intestinal tract; however, they cause CNS, cardiovascular, hepatic, and muscular diseases.
 They get to the target tissues by hematogenous dissemination through blood hence circulating antibodies will protect against disease but have no effect on infection.

The German word "pech" can be translated "bad luck". It can also serve as a mnemonic for the Enteroviruses:

P = _____

E = _____

C = _____

H = _____

Non A/non B hepatitis is the most common cause of transfusion-induced hepatitis; this is because most of the blood used in hospitals has been screened for Hepatitis B. Hepatitis A is the most common hepatitis virus; why isn't it the number 1 cause of post-transfusion hepatitis?
 [see hepatitis section for answer]

The table below is a helpful way to group the viruses. There are 6 families of DNA-containing viruses, Herpes, Hepadna, Adeno, Papova, Pox and Parvo (The HHAPPPy viruses). If one can remember these and the generalities associated with the DNA viruses, then any other virus will be the opposite. As nothing is ever that simple, the table also contains the exceptions to that rule, e.g., if all DNA viruses are Double stranded and Naked, then the RNA viruses should all be single stranded and enveloped; and they are with the exception of the REO (dsRNA) and Picorna (naked RNA) as noted in the table. The nucleic acid of all viruses is linear except for two Hepatitis viruses, B and D, and the Papovaviruses.

VIRUS CLASSIFICATION

Virus Type	Generalities	Exceptions
DNA Viruses	Double Stranded	Parvo
Herpes Hepadna Adeno Papova Pox Parvo	Naked	Herpes, HBV and Pox
	Nuclear site for Replication	Pox
	Icosahedral (cubic) symmetry	Pox (complex)

RNA Viruses*	Single Stranded	REO
Paramyxo Toga Picorna Corona Rhabdo Orthomyxo Arena Bunya Retro REO Flavi	Enveloped	REO and Picorna
	Helical symmetry	REO, Picorna, Retro and Toga
	Cytoplasmic site for replication	Orthomyxo and Retro (nuclear + cytoplasmic)

* The first 5 viruses listed are polycistronic single RNA strands; the remaining viruses have segmented genomes

VIRAL REPLICATION

STEPS	ACTIVITY	
1. Adsorption	-virus attaches to specific receptors on cell membrane -interaction is, at first, reversible, then becomes irreversible	The first step in viral replication is
2. Penetration	-virus particle is actively taken up by cell through a process called pinocytosis or phagocytosis	_____. Antibody to viral <u>capsid/nucleic acid</u>
3. Uncoating	-takes place at cell membrane or vesicles -viral nucleic acid is released inside of cell by cell host enzymes	blocks this process.
4. Intracellular replication of viral components		
A. RNA viruses	-picorna and toga-viruses - the genome is +RNA and serves as mRNA	Early viral proteins are _____
	-others (e.g., myxo [ortho & para], rhabdo) carry viral RNA dependent RNA polymerase which synthesizes +mRNA from viral -RNA strands.	_____ _____; late proteins are _____
	-early proteins are enzymes for viral RNA synthesis or inhibitors of cellular synthetic events.	_____
	-late proteins are viral structural proteins and assembly proteins synthesized in response to the viral genome	_____.
B. DNA viruses		
1. RNA synthesis	-host cell supplies transcriptase, pox has its own DNA dependent RNA polymerase	
2. Early protein synthesis	-synthesis of enzymes for DNA synthesis, tumor antigens, etc.	

3. Viral DNA	—many new copies of viral DNA synthesis

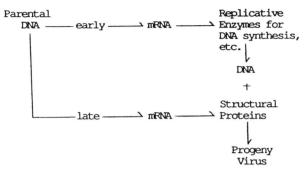

4. Late protein synthesis	—viral capsid proteins(structural)

5. Assembly:	—newly synthesized viral nucleic acid and protein assembled inside cell —viral envelope added (usually from cell membrane) —new viruses released from cell by budding or lysis

6. Effects of Viruses on Cells	—lytic viruses inhibit cell RNA, DNA, protein synthesis —tumor viruses transform cells —latent viruses (herpes) probably do not alter host cell greatly

The template for early proteins in a Herpes infected cell is provided by <u>viral RNA/viral DNA via newly synthesized RNA.</u>

REPLICATION OF SPECIFIC RNA VIRUSES

1. <u>Picorna Corona Togavirus</u> ex. polio rubella WEE	—viral RNA is single stranded piece of messenger RNA (+mRNA) —naked viral RNA can infect cells —viral RNA (+mRNA) gets to polysomes to make new viral proteins —new proteins made as one long protein, then cleaved to viral specific proteins —replicase (RNA-dependent RNA polymerase), an enzyme which copies +mRNA and makes a negative strand of mRNA —the —mRNA is then used as template to make new viral RNA (+mRNA)

Replication of Positive Stranded RNA Viruses

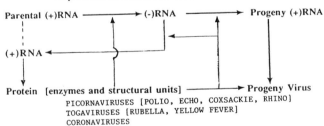

PICORNAVIRUSES [POLIO, ECHO, COXSACKIE, RHINO]
TOGAVIRUSES [RUBELLA, YELLOW FEVER]
CORONAVIRUSES

The template for poliovirus RNA is <u>+mRNA/—mRNA.</u>

29

2. Orthomyxovirus
   (influenza virus)
   - viral RNA is
     fragmented into 8
     pieces of (-mRNA)
   - virus carries into
     cell a transcriptase
     enzyme (RNA dependent
     RNA polymerase)
   - transcriptase copies
     (-mRNA) to make
     (+mRNA) for viral
     proteins
   - (+mRNA) is also
     template for new
     viral (-mRNA)

3. Paramyxoviruses and Rhabdoviruses
   (mumps, measles, rabies)
   - viral RNA is
     single-stranded
     (-mRNA), not
     segmented
   - virus carries
     transcriptase like
     the influenza virus;
     similar replication
     cycle

4. Diplornavirus
   (reovirus and rotovirus)
   - viral RNA is double-
     stranded and composed
     of ten fragments
   - virus carries
     transcriptase

5. Retroviruses
   (RNA tumor virses)
   - viral RNA is single
     stranded
   - virus carries reverse
     transcriptase (RNA-
     dependent DNA poly-
     merase)
   - transcriptase copies
     viral RNA into DNA
   - DNA is integrated into
     host genome and serves
     as template for new
     viral RNA

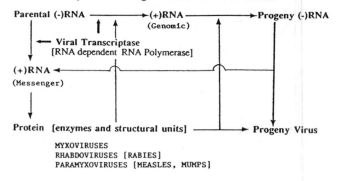

Replication of Negative Stranded RNA Viruses

MYXOVIRUSES
RHABDOVIRUSES [RABIES]
PARAMYXOVIRUSES [MEASLES, MUMPS]

The RNA dependent RNA polymerase found in
influenza virus is also called

_____ ;

it converts -RNA into +RNA template for

protein synthesis.

Replication of Double Stranded RNA Viruses
REO & ROTAVIRUSES

The template for mumps capsid is provided

for by viral RNA/newly synthesized RNA.

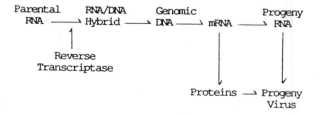

Replication of Retroviruses

30

REPLICATION OF SPECIFIC DNA VIRUSES

1. Herpesvirus
   -replicates inside
   nucleus
   -viral envelope
   obtained from
   nuclear membrane

   RNA dependent RNA polymerase is a part
   of the following viruses

   1. _____

2. Adenovirus
   -replicates inside
   nucleus

   2. _____

3. Poxvirus
   -replicates in cyto-
   plasm; complex
   -virus carries many
   enzymes into cell

   3. _____

   4. _____

4. Papovavirus
   -replicates in
   nucleus, circular DNA

VIRAL ENZYMES

VIRUS	ENZYMES
Negative RNA ex orthomyxo paramyxxo rhabdo	RNA polymerase
Retrovirus	Reverse transcriptase RNAse H [breaks down RNA in RNA-DNA strand] Polynucleotide ligase [closes DNA breaks]
Pox	More than a dozen e. g., DNA-dependent RNA polymerase RNA methylase DNAse
Herpes	Thymidine kinase* DNA polymerase*
Reoviruses including Roto	RNA polymerase
Hepatitis B	DNA-dependent DNA polymerase Protein kinases

* produced in cell not brought in with virion

31

ANTIVIRAL AGENTS

INTERFERENCE WITH VIRAL REPLICATION

1. Interferon (IFN)
   -a group of proteins made by cells in response to viruses, synthetic nucleotides (poly r:IC), foreign cells that interferes with viral replication

   Interferon produced by a macrophage would be an alpha/beta interferon

   IFN species
   leukocyte (alpha), fibroblast (beta), lymphocyte (gamma/immune)
   -cell genome has information for IFN: if one inhibits cell metabolism with actinomycin D, no IFN produced
   -IFN induces cells to make products which inhibit viral or foreign cell replication
   -IFN released from cells, spreads to other cells and induces new IFN

   Interferon is effective against

   A. DNA viruses

   B. RNA viruses

   C. Both

   D. Neither

   (answer at bottom of page)

   IFN induced products
   1. **2'5'A synthetase** which polymerizes ATP into an oligonucleotide that activates RNAse L which degrades viral RNA
   2. **eIF-2α kinase** which autophosphorylates in the presence of dsRNA. The modified kinase then phosphorylates eukaryotic initiation factor-2 (eIF-2) which inhibits viral mRNA translation

   Biologic Activities of interferon
   1. antiviral
   2. Inhibition of cell growth
   3. Immune modulation
      a. NK
      b. ADCC
      c. macrophage activation

   Interferon inhibits viral replication by inducing cellular production of

   1. _____

   2. _____

   both of which interfere with viral mRNA activity.

2. Specific Antibody
   1. IgG, A, M
   2. Neutralize by interfering with the functions of viral capsid or envelop proteins. The antibodies block - absorption
                    - penetration
                    - uncoating (rare)

   (answer = C)

3. CHEMICAL INHIBITORS

a. **Amantidine** and **rimantidine** both inhibit viral uncoating that follows viral entry into the cytoplasm of the cell. They may also interfere with transcription of viral RNA. They are used against influenza strain A viruses; strain B is resistant.

b. **Idoxuridine** and **trifluorothymidine** are halogenated pyrimidines that are able to block DNA synthesis because they are incorporated into DNA in the place of thymidine. They are very toxic and used mainly against herpetic keratitis.

c. **Adenine arabinoside** (Ara-A) inhibits DNA viruses, especially Herpes. It must be phosphorylated intracellularly before it becomes an inhibitor for **DNA polymerase**. Less toxic than idoxuridine.

d. **Dideoxycytidine** and **dideoxyinosine** are phosphorylated intracellularly to their triphosphate form and are then able to block viral reverse transcriptase, thus interfering with **HIV** replication.

e. **Acyclovir** is very active against Herpes simplex, less so against zoster and Epstein Barr viruses and inactive vs cytomegalovirus. It is phosphorylated intracytoplasmically by **viral thymidine kinase** (which explains its spectrum of activity) into a monophosphate which is further phosphorylated by cellular kinase to the active triphosphate form which binds to and inhibits viral **DNA polymerase**.

f. **Gancyclovir** is an analog of acyclovir that is active against all herpes viruses. It is used primarily for **cytomegaloviral infections**; this virus does not encode a thymidine kinase and hence is resistant to acyclovir. The cellular kinases phosphorylate gancyclovir to its active form that blocks DNA polymerase. There is significant toxicity associated with gancyclovir; it suppresses spermatogenesis, bone marrow precursors, and gut epithelium.

g. **Azidothymidine** inhibits **HIV** replication by inhibiting reverse transcriptase and causing termination of viral DNA strand elongation. It is phosphorylated by cellular kinases to its active triphosphate form.

h. **Ribavirin** is active against both DNA and RNA viruses. It interferes with viral nucleic acid synthesis by unclear mechanisms. It is used in aerosol form to treat **Respiratory Syncytial Viral infections** in infants.

Antiviral drugs activated in vivo by cellular kinase enzymes that phosphorylate the drug to an active form include

1. _____

2. _____

3. _____

4. _____

5. _____

The DOC (drug of choice) for RSV is

_____.

The DOC for Herpes simplex is

_____.

Amantadine is used to treat _____.

HIV infections can be treated with

1. _____

VIRAL IMMUNOTHERAPY AND PROPHYLAXIS

I. Active, Artificial Immunity

A. Recommended for all persons in US

Disease	Condition of Vaccine
1. Rubella*	live attenuated
2. Measles*	live attenuated
3. Mumps*	live attenuated
4. Polio	
(Sabin)**	live attenuated
(Salk)**	inactive

> Live viral vaccines are NOT recommended for immunosuppressed individuals

B. Recommended for special conditions (epidemic, military, travel, exposure)

Disease	Condition of Vaccine
1. Rabies***	inactive
2. Yellow Fever	live attenuated
3. Influenza**	inactive
4. Adenovirus**	active
5. Togavirus	inactive
6. Chickenpox	live attenuated
7. Hepatitis B	inactive

*May be combined; all are a single anti-
genic type
**May be polyvalent
***Usually given with immune serum

II. PASSIVE, ARTIFICIAL IMMUNITY-use of immune serum or gamma globulin. Used only under special circumstances.

1. Rabies	4. Rubeola
2. Rubella	5. Mumps
3. Hepatitis A and B	6. Chicken Pox
	7. Polio

This type of treatment may be effective in disease prevention; it is of little value after onset of disease.

III. New approaches to acquired immunity is the use of
1. viral subunit particles
2. synthesis of viral peptides:
   a. in bacteria via cDNA technology
   b. by other, non-pathogenic hybrid viruses (e.g. vaccinia)

MMR vaccine combination consists of

1. _____

2. _____

3. _____

> Live viral vaccines induce immunity of long duration.

Polyvalent viral vaccines include

1. _____

2. _____

3. _____

34

REVIEW STATEMENTS

These should be used to strengthen and expand you understanding of Microbial Physiology. The statements are "factoids" that may help in the STEP 1 exam. You may wish to develop your own list to expand your knowledge base. If you have a spare sheet of paper available, white down the correct statement for every question you miss in going through review exams. This way you can avoid marking on the review exam (so you can use it again) and still have captured that fact for future review.

Flagella are the organelles responsible for motility of bacteria. Their direction of rotation controls movement; counterclockwise=forward (positive) chemotaxis.

Pili are short hair-like protein structures which occur on the surface of bacteria. Some, for example, those that occur on the gonococcus, are thought to be associated with the **adherence** of the organism to host cells. The sex pilus, which is found only in male strains of bacteria, is involved in **conjugation**.

Capsules of most species of bacteria are composed of **carbohydrate**, with the exception of *Bacillus anthracis*, which has a capsule composed of poly-D glutamic acid. In many pathogenic microorganisms the capsule **inhibits phagocytosis.**

Three kinds of proteins are associated with the **cytoplasmic membrane** of bacteria. They include **biosynthetic enzymes, transport proteins** and **cytochrome enzymes,** which serve the following functions in the cell: synthesis of external layers of the cell, transport of water-soluble materials into the cytoplasm, and electron transport activities, respectively.

Spores are highly resistant to deleterious agents in the environment, probably because of the content of **keratin-like proteins** in the spore coat, and their low metabolic rate.

The **periplasmic space** and outer layer are unique to the Gram negative bacteria, as are **porin channels** in the outer membrane. **Teichoic acids** are unique to Gram positive microorganisms.

Bacterial resistance to antibiotics is usually conferred by **plasmids** (R factors) which induce **production of enzymes** with modify the antibiotic.

A complication of **clindamycin** therapy is **enterocolitis** caused by *Clostridium difficile.*

Chloramphenicol is useful in the treatment of typhoid fever and *Haemophilus influenzae* meningitis.

Penicillin and **cephalosporin** inhibit **transpeptidation**, the final reaction of mucopeptide synthesis. Bacterial resistance to these two antibiotics is usually the result of a β-**lactamase**, whose production is governed by a **plasmid.** Penicillin-destroying enzymes from Gram positive bacteria are relatively inactive against 2nd and 3rd generation cephalosporins.

Rifampin inhibits the action of DNA dependent RNA polymerase by binding to the polymerase.

Sulfonamides are **bacteriostatic** drugs which inhibit the condensation of pteridine pyrophosphate with PABA: they block dihydrofolate synthetase; **trimethoprim** blocks the action of dihydrofolate reductase. An analog of PABA which has a similar mechanism of action is **para-amino salicylic acid**, which is used in the treatment of tuberculosis. Sulfanilamide is relatively non-toxic for humans because we are unable to synthesize **folic acid.**

Streptomycin causes damage to the eighth cranial nerve.

Tetracyclines are broad spectrum agents that bind the 30S ribosome and inhibit binding of aminoacyl tRNA.

Chloramphenicol and the **tetracyclines** are both broad specrum antibiotics which inhibit protein synthesis; they differ in that chloramphenicol attaches to the 50S ribosomal subunit while tetracyclines attach to the 30S subunit. Chloramphenicol interferes with protein synthesis by inhibiting peptide bond formation (**peptidyl transferase**).

Cessation of bacterial growth is caused by toxic metabolic end products, unfavorable pH, and nutrient exhaustion.

Methicillin and **oxacillin** are used for penicillin-resistant strains of bacteria.

Lipid A, core and O antigen are all parts of lipopolysaccharide(endotoxin); **lipid A is toxic**.

Drugs which affect the 30S ribosome are the **aminoglycosides** and **tetracyclines**.

D-Cycloserine, vancomycin and **bacitracin** are all inhibitors of peptidoglycan synthesis.

Surfactants, particularly **cationic detergents** (e.g., quaternary compounds such as zephiran) act by **disrupting the cell membrane** or viral envelop.

Phenol is both a detergent and an effective protein denaturant. **Alcohols** such as ethanol and isopropyl alcohol also are bactericidal due to **protein denaturant** activity.

Pseudomonads are highly **resistant to antibiotics** because 1) their porin channels limit the passage of water soluble molecules, and 2) highly active antibiotic inactivating enzymes are produced by these organisms.

Metronidazole is useful against *Giardia*, *Trichomonas* and anaerobic bacteria. It is coverted to its active form inside the parasite by low redox potential compounds such as ferredoxin.

The **protein coat** (capsid) of true viruses functions to **maintain infectivity** of nucleic acid in the extracellular state, serves as an antigen in **vaccines,** and **aids in the penetration** of virions into susceptible cells. **Cell susceptibility** range of a virus is determined by surface protein units of the capsid or envelope

One of the first events which occurs after a virulent virus infects a cell is **cessation of host cell macromolecular biosynthesis.**

IUDR (5 iodo-2' deoxyuridine) is incorporated into viral DNA to produce faulty nucleic acid.

The **picornaviruses** are single strands of (+) RNA. During replication replicative intermediates (RI=double stranded RNA; a +RNA and a -RNA) are formed by the enzyme **replicase**. Orthomyxoviruses and paramyxoviruses also have an RI; however, these viruses have a (-) RNA as the parental type. Viral transcriptase (**RNA dependent RNA polymerase**) makes (+) RNA used as mRNA for protein synthesis. **Orthomyxoviruses** have eight distinct (-) RNA strands; **paramyxo's** only have one. **Reovirus** RNA is double stranded RNA which exists in 10 distinct segments.

The capsid proteins in the **progeny of a hybrid virus** (e.g.polio RNA in a coxsackie capsid) will be encoded by the genetic information of the nucleic acid donor.

Replication of **HIV** would be blocked by inhibitors of **DNA-dependent RNA polymerase.**

Varicella virus gets its envelop from the **nuclear** membrane.

Picornaviruses use specific **viral proteases** to produce mature **viral proteins** from precursor polyproteins.

Viral envelopes are important for viral **adsorption and entry** into cells.

Viral uncoating occurs after the virus has gained entry into the cell.

Acyclovir is effective against several **Herpes viruses**; it is activated in the cell by **phosphorylation** catalyzed by a **virally-encoded enzyme.**

Ganciclovir is the drug of choice for **cytomegalovirus**

Ribavirin by aerosol route is the recommended therapy for **Respiratory Syncytial Virus** infection in neonates.

36

MICROBIAL PHYSIOLOGY REVIEW EXAM

SELECT THE SINGLE BEST COMPLETION FOR EACH QUESTION .

1. If a composite virus contains the RNA from Hepatitis A and the capsid of Hepatitis C

    A. only Hepatitis C progeny would be formed
    B. the composite virus would reproduce itself to form new composite virus
    C. the host-cell range of the composite virus would be the same as that of Hepatitis A
    D. the host-cell range of the progeny would be the same as that of Hepatitis A
    E. the host cell range of the progeny would be the same as that of Hepatitis C

2. Cytomegalovirus infections are treated most efficiently with

    A. acyclovir.
    B. amantadine.
    C. azidothymidine
    D. ganciclovir.
    E. ribavirin.

3. *Staphylococcus aureus* isolated from hospitals is usually penicillin resistant whereas *S. aureus* isolated from the community at large is usually penicillin sensitive. The reason for this difference is

    A. hospital personnel usually are colonized with penicillin-sensitive strains.
    B. hospital strains mutate forming penicillin-resistant strains which survive better than sensitive strains.
    C. hospital strains acquire a plasmid which carries the structural gene for penicillinase.
    D. non-hospital strains do not form β-lactamase because it is an inducible enzyme which is only formed in the presence of penicillin.

4. A structure which contains lipid A, core polysaccharide and O antigen would occur in an organism

    A. with a periplasmic space.
    B. with ribitol teichoic acid in its cell wall.
    C. which forms spores.
    D. which is Gram positive.
    E. with flagella.

5. Ribavirin

    A. is best used together with AZT to treat AIDS.
    B. inhibits viral attachment.
    C. must must be phosphorylated intracellularly to be active.
    D. is used in aerosol form to treat respiratory syncytial virus infections in infants.

6. A β–lactamase inhibitor that can be co-administered with penicillin to render a penicillin resistant Staphylococcus species susceptible to the antibiotic is

    A. lysozyme.
    B. clavulanic acid.
    C. cephalosporinase.
    D. penicillin-binding protein.

7. What is the basis of the specific toxicity of ketoconazole?

    A. Bacteria lack sterols in their membranes
    B. The primary sterol in fungal membranes is ergosterol
    C. The presence of the endo-plasmic reticulum in mammalian cells
    D. Humans require folic acid preformed

8. N-acetyl glucosamine and N-acetylmuramic acid are fundamental building blocks for growth. They are a part of which component of the bacterial cell?

A. outer membrane.
B. inner membrane.
C. lipopolysaccharide.
D. peptidoglycan.
E. capsule.

9. Most disinfectants eliminate infectious organisms by

A. bacteristatic mechanisms
B. reducing the microbial flora to a federally accepted level.
C. killing the vegetative cells.
D. killing vegetative cells and spores.

10. Tetracyclines are useful drugs which

A. prevent RNA synthesis.
B. are bactericidal.
C. prevent binding of aminoacyl tRNA to the 30S ribosome.
D. bind to the L12 subunit of the 50S ribosome.

11. Introduction of a naked viral genome in the cytoplasm is infectious (leads to a productive infection) with which virus?

A. adenovirus
B. HIV
C. poliovirus
D. parvovirus
E. mumps virus

12. Several antivirals are nucleotide analogs, including both:

A. IUdR and acyclovir
B. acyclovir and interferon
C. amantadine and azidothymidine
D. cyclophosphamide and vidarabine

13. Interferon

A. interferes directly with translation of viral RNA.
B. blocks penetration of viruses into susceptible cells.
C. induces host cells to produce antiviral proteins that interfere with translation of viral messenger RNA.
D. interferes with viral absorption onto cell membranes.

14. Which three antibiotics bind the bacterial 50s ribosome?

A. Tetracycline, streptomycin and bacitracin
B. Erythromycin, chloramphenicol and lincomycin
C. Tobramycin, gentamicin and amikacin
D. Bacitracin, vancomycin and D-cycloserine

15. A unique feature of eucaryotic cells that is not found in procaryotic cells is a

A. nuclear membrane.
B. periplasm.
C. peptidoglycan layer.
D. 70s ribosome.

16. Incorporation of uracil into bacterial nucleic acids would be inhibited by which of the following antimicrobials?

A. Penicillin
B. Streptomycin
C. Chloramphenicol
D. Rifampin
E. Tetracycline

17. The outer membrane of a Gram negative bacteria is resistant to the action of detergents largely due to the presence of

A. lipoteichoic acids.
B. phosphotidyl inositol.
C. cholesterol and ergosterol.
D. lipoprotein and lipopolysaccharide.
E. glycoproteins and the capsule.

18. A patient develops a fever, goes into shock and dies in the hospital. Upon performing a blood culture you find that the paitent had a Gram negative sepsis. What is the likely cause of the paitent's fever and subsequent demise?

A. Peptidoglycan components that are released into the blood
B. The presence of pili on the bacterial cell
C. The presence of lipopolysaccharide in the outer membrane
D. The release of lipoprotein by the bacterial cell on autolysis

19. The membrane bound chemoreceptors of the chemotactic system undergo what type of modification which is the trigger for chemotaxis?

    A. phosphorylation
    B. methylation
    C. acetylation
    D. dephosphorylation
    E. proteolytic cleavage

20. What antifungal agent interferes with the biosynthesis of ergosterol?

    A. Amphotericin B
    B. Ketoconazole
    C. Polymyxin
    D. Nystatin
    E. potassium Iodide

21. Cycloserine is a water soluble antibiotic with a molecular weight of 102. You would predict that it would

    A. arrive in the periplasmic space by diffusion through the porin pores of the outer membrane.
    B. arrieve in the periplasmic space by diffusion through the phopholipid region of the outer membrane.
    C. be transported through the cell membrane by the phosphotransferase system.
    D. Pass through the cell membrane by simple diffusion.
    E. probably not pass through the cell membrane

22. Chloramphenicol is more effective against prokaryotes than eukaryotes because it

    A. inhibits prokaryotic DNA-directed RNA polymerase.
    B. inhibits protein synthesis by 70S, but not by 80S ribosomes.
    C. activates a cell wall autolysin.
    D. causes misreading of UUU codon in mRNA.
    E. inhibits DNA synthesis by prokaryotes.

23. Streptomycin

    A. inhibits peptidyl transferase.
    B. prevents initiation of protein synthesis by ribosomes of prokaryotes.
    C. disrupts cell membranes which contain sterols.
    D. binds to 50S ribosomes such that it inhibits peptide bond formation.
    E. prevents binding of mRNA to the ribosome.

24. One important reason why trimethoprim and sulfamethoxazole together are more effective against bacteria than the sum of their individual activities is because

    A. both inhibit dihydropteroic acid synthetase.
    B. both inhibit dihydrofolate reductase.
    C. trimethoprim is bacteristatic and sulfamethaxazole is bactericidal.
    D. trimethoprim inhibits cell wall synthesis and sulfamethoxazole inhibits folic acid synthesis.
    E. both inhibit folic acid synthesis, but inhibit different steps.

25. During herpesvirus replication:

    A. Viral capsid proteins mediate cell attachment
    B. Viral regulatory proteins and enzymes are made in immediate early phase
    C. Late transcription takes place in the cytoplasm
    D. DNA is replicated by host cell DNA polymerase

26. Prokaryotes contain which of the following structures?

    A. Nuclear membrane
    B. Histones
    C. Endoplasmic reticulum
    D. Ribosomes
    E. Mitochondria

27. Virus envelopes

   A. Provide protection for viruses during tansit through the stomach and intestine.
   B. contain the transcriptases necessary for production of mRNA in host cells.
   C. contain subunits called capsomeres and protomers.
   D. are important for virus adsorption and entry into cells.

28. During adenovirus replication

   A. Capsid proteins attach to receptors on the nuclear membrane
   B. Viral DNA is replicated by cellular DNA polymerase
   C. Late and early transcription takes place in the cytoplasm
   D. Capsid proteins are made during immediate early phase

29. A structure which contains lipid A, core polysaccharide and O antigen would occur in an organism

   A. with a periplasmic space.
   B. with ribitol teichoic acid in its cell wall.
   C. which forms spores.
   D. which is Gram positive.
   E. with flagella.

30. Actinomycin D selectively blocks DNA dependent RNA polymerases. This drug would be expected to inhibit which of the following viruses?

   A. Hepatitis A virus.
   B. Hepatitis E virus.
   C. Retrovirus.
   D. Togavirus.

DIRECTIONS (ITEMS 31-38): Each of the numbered items or incomplete statements in this section is negatively phrased, as indicated by a capitalized word such as **NOT, LEAST,** or **EXCEPT**. Select the **ONE** lettered answer or completion that is **BEST** in each case and fill in the circle containing the corresponding letter on the answer sheet.

31. All of the following antiviral agents would be effective against DNA viruses **EXCEPT**

   A. interferon.
   B. amantadine.
   C. iododeoxyuridine.
   D. ribavirin.
   E. adenosine arabinoside.

32. All of the following are properties of acyclovir **EXCEPT**

   A. effective in inhibiting Herpesvirus replication.
   B. can be administered orally and intravenously.
   C. blocks penetration of virus into host cells.
   D. activity based upon viral thymidine kinase.

33. Resistance to tetracycline is a common trait in bacteria largely due to the fact that tetracycline is used to promote weight gain in beef cattle and it is an over-the-counter drug in most third world countries. Therefore many different mechanisms of resistance to tetracycline have evolved in the bacteria. What is **NOT** a mechanism of resistance to tetracycline?

   A. Efflux of tetracycline from the cell by a specific transport protein
   B. Modification of ribosomes so the drug will not bind
   C. The presence of porin channels in the outer membrane
   D. Modification of tetracycline by a specific enzyme that inactivates it

34. If you were treating a patient with a Mycoplasma pneumonia what antibiotic would you clearly **NOT** use?

   A. streptomycin
   B. erythromycin
   C. tetracycline
   D. penicillin

35. Actinomycin D selectively blocks DNA dependent RNA polymerases. This drug would be expected to inhibit all of the following **EXCEPT**

   A. Polyomavirus.
   B. Hepatitis B virus.
   C. Togavirus.
   D. Retrovirus.

36. All of the following are true about the effect of penicillin G on *Streptococcus pneumoniae* **EXCEPT**

   A. most pronounced when added during the exponential phase of growth.

   B. results in death of the streptococci.
   C. prevent formation of peptidoglycan cross links.
   D. depends on the presence of an autolysin.
   E. dissolves the outer membrane of the cell.

37. If you were treating a patient with a *Mycoplasma* pneumonia, what antibiotic would you clearly **NOT** use?

   A. Streptomycin
   B. Erythromycin
   C. Rifampicin
   D. Chloramphenicol
   E. Penicillin

38. All of the following antiviral agent would be effective against DNA viruses **EXCEPT**

   A. interferon.
   B. amantadine.
   C. iododeoxyuridine.
   D. ribavirin.
   E. adenosine arabinoside.

Questions 39-40
The antibiotic pictured is penicillin. Select the area of the molecule that best matches each statement below

39. In a penicillin resistant *Staphylococcus aureus*, the antibiotic is inactivated by hydrolysis at which point?

40. Resistance to the action of penicillinase, as well as changes in the spectrum of sensitivity of microbes to the antibiotic, is conferred by modification of the above molecule at what site?

41

| MATCH THE THERAPEUTIC AGENT WITH THE PATIENT DESCRIBED BELOW. |
| AN ANSWER MAY BE USE MORE THAN ONCE, OR NOT AT ALL. |

A.	Penicillin	G.	Isoniazid
B.	Streptomycin	H.	Erythromycin
C.	Oxacillin	I.	Trimethoprim-sulfamethoxazole
D.	Metronidazole	J.	Clavulanic acid
E.	Ribavirin	K.	Azidothymidine
F.	Acyclovir	L.	Flucytosine

41. This 12 year old young lady has cardiac abnormalities consistent with Rheumatic carditis. Three weeks following a routine visit to her oral hygienist, she develops fever and chills. She develops splinter hemorrhages in her nail beds, and is hospitalized with a diagnosis of subacute bacterial endocarditis.

42. A Marine sargent reports to the Infirmary with a low grade fever and a non-productive cough. Her serum agglutinates Streptococcus strain MG.

43 A young kindergarten student develops otitis media after a ski trip with her family. Culture yielded a gram positive coccus in short chains which grew on blood agar with alpha hemolysis. Growth was inhibited by optochin.

44. A 24 year old third year Medical student came to the student health service for a check-up after a serious exposure to an AIDS patient with tuberculosis. His lungs were clear to auscultation; no lesions were seen on X-ray. His ppd skin test was negative; however on re-testing 3 weeks later a reaction measuring 14 mm of induration was observed.

45. A 14 week old infant is admitted to the hospital for a severe respiratory infection. Histological examination of exfoliated cells in repiratory secretions reveals numberous syncytial masses.

46. A 12 year old girl scout has been hospitalized with a diagnosis of meningitis. The spinal fluid contains numerous PMNs and gram negative coccal forms. The organism is cultured on Thayer Martin medium and is found to ferment both glucose and maltose.

47. This three year old presents with a high fever and a stiff neck. Spinal fluid analysis reveals an elevated opening pressure, pleocytosis, a decrease in glucose content (20% of blood glucose levels), increased levels of immunoglobulins, and *H. influenzae* type b capsular carbohydrate antigen.

48. This 19 year old pom pom girl has moderate flu-like symptoms and a sore throat. Her serum contains antibodies that agglutinate sheep erythrocytes.

49. The child brought to the hospital Emergency room is in great respiratory distress. She has a fever of 40.2 C and is producing blood tinged sputum. A gram stain of the sputum reveals numerous neutrophils and gram positive cocci in random clusters.

50. This 49 year old pidgeon breeder has been experiencing intermittent frontal headaches and malaise. His wife has noted that he seems disoriented and irrational at times. Cerebrospinal fluid contains numerous lymphocytes and a few phagocytic cells containing budding yeast cells.

KEY

1. D	11. C	21. A	31. B	41. A
2. D	12. A	22. B	32. C	42. A
3. C	13. C	23. B	33. C	43. A
4. A	14. B	24. E	34. D	44. E
5. D	15. A	25. B	35. C	45. E.
6. B	16. D	26. D	36. E	46. A
7. B	17. D	27. D	37. E	47. B
8. D	18. C	28. A	38. B	48. F
9. C	19. B	29. A	39. D	49. C
10. C	20. B	30. C	40. E	50. L

MICROBIAL GENETICS

MUTATIONS

The term mutation refers to an abrupt and usually stably inherited change in properties of an organism. Mutations can occur either spontaneously, or may be induced by a mutagen. (see table, pg. 47)

Mutation in Populations

The proportion of mutants in a given population of cells is called the mutant frequency. The probability that a mutation will occur during a particular time interval, such as the generation time, is the mutation rate, and is expressed as a mutation per cell, per division.

Selection of Mutants

Wild type is the designation given to strains as they are found in nature, or to certain laboratory standard strains. Mutants, called auxotrophs, have an additional nutritional requirement. Markers are other detectable mutations with a distinctive observable effect on the organism serving to mark the chromosome at the locus at which it occurs. Such markers include colony morphology, fermentation patterns and antibiotic resistance.

Point Mutations

Point mutations may occur as a result of a base pair substitution in the specific nucleotide sequence of a gene. When one purine on a chain replaces another purine, and when the pyrimidine on the other chain is replaced by a different pyrimidine, the substitution is called a transition.

Transversions occur when a purine in a DNA chain is replaced by a pyrimidine, and when the pyrimidine on the other chain is replaced by a purine.

Transitions may be produced by agents such as 5-bromouracil or 2-aminopurine. Alkylating agents such as ethylethane-

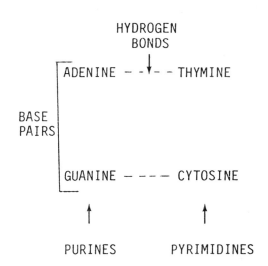

DEFINE THE FOLLOWING POINT MUTATIONS
(Answers on next page)

1. GC changes to AT

2. GC changes to TA

3. CG changes to AT

4. TA changes to GC

sulfonate also cause transitions. Nitrous acid oxidatively deaminates the amino-substituted bases; adenine, guanine, and cytosine.

A missense mutation occurs when the above substitution occurs and the triplet code is altered such that a different amino acid is inserted into the protein. The product may be inactive or only partially active.

A nonsense mutation occurs when the above substitution occurs and the triplet code is altered such that a chain termination codon (UAG, UAA, or UGA) appears.

Frameshift mutations are those mutations which result in an addition or deletion of a nucleotide into a sequence of mRNA cause a reading frameshift of the trinucleotide sequences. Frameshift mutations may result in an addition or deletion of one, two, four or five nucleotides, all of which result in a shift of the reading frame. Frameshift mutations are known to be caused by a group of polycyclic compounds called acridines (e.g., proflavin). Acridines are capable of strong binding to DNA by intercalation between adjacent base pairs.

Deletions

Mutations resulting in the loss of large segments of DNA, covering from one to several genes, are referred to as deletions. Deletions can occur spontaneously, or may be induced by X-rays, UV Light, or treatment with nitrous acid.

Carcinogenic compounds have been found to be mutagens once they are activated by liver microsomal oxidases. In the activated state, as epoxides, these agents act preferentially as frameshift mutagens. Chemical mutagens, particularly those of the frameshift variety, may be important factors in carcinogenesis.

Define the following mutations, identify a suitable mutagen, and describe the consequences of the mutation. Remember, nonsense codons are UAG, UAA, UGA.

(answers on next page)

Wild type gene=AUG-ACC-UGG-UCA-CCA-TTT-AAT-

Auxotroph #1=AUG-ACT-UGG-UCA-CCA-TTT-AAT-

Auxotroph #2=AUG-ACC-UGA-GUC-ACC-ATT-TAA-T

Auxotroph #3=AUG-ACC-UUC-ACC-ATT-TAA-T

Auxotroph #4=UAG-ATT

Answers to point mutations question

1 = transition
2 = transversion
3 = transversion
4 = transversion

44

RECOMBINATION

Recombination is the formation of a new genotype by reassortment of genes following a genetic cross. It involves a structural change due to the crossing over, or exchange of genetic material between two different, but homologous chromosomes; significant sequence homology is required. Only a portion of the donor chromosome is added to the recipient to form a partial diploid. Significant sequence homology must exist before recombination can take place.

Model of Recombination: The Breakage and Reunion model of recombination proposes that the chromosomes break and are reunited such that each progeny contains genetic material from both parents. This model is supported by the observation that recombination can occur without DNA synthesis. Reciprocal recombination is the rule, however, on occasion, the recombinant is unidirectional (progeny contains genes from one parent but the 2nd reunion does not occur).

COMPLEMENTATION

Complementation is the process by which two recessive mutations can supply each other's deficiency to produce a wild type phenotype. It is another method of genetic analysis used to determine whether two mutants, apparently defective in the same way, are defective in the same gene. It should not be confused with recombination which deals with structural changes between genes. Two types of complementation are known to occur.

Intergenic complementation occurs with genes specifying proteins consisting of two or more nonidentical polypeptides.

Intragenic complementation occurs with genes specifying multimeric proteins consisting of two or more identical polypeptides.

```
Transferred chromosomal fragments
cannot replicate unless they are
integrated into the recipient DNA
(e.g. in transformation and some
conjugation events).
```

Types of Recombination

A. Legitimate (Generalized)

Host cell enzymes that are involved include:
Rec A = Proteolytic and ATPase activities
Rec BC = Endonuclease, exonuclease
Nucleases
DNA polymerase
DNA ligase

B. Nonhomologous (or illegitimate)

Independent of Rec A gene function
e.g. = Transposon insertion, and certain phage mediated events.

Answers to Auxotroph questions

1= Transition; 5-bromouracil; missense mutation-protein may or may not lose function
2= Frameshift by insertion; acridine orange or proflavin; nonsense mutation-protein loses function due to premature chain termination
3= Frameshift by deletion; acridine dyes; missense mutation-usually loss of protein function
4= Deletion of larger segment of DNA:irradiation, nitrous acid or bi-functional alkylating agent; protein loses function

45

SUPPRESSION

The effects of a harmful mutation in an organism may be reversed to yield the wild type phenotype. When this occurs there may be a true back mutation to the original genotype, or the genetic code may be misread leaving the original mutation unchanged. When the effects of a primary mutation are eliminated by altering the translation process, the phenomenon is called suppression. Two types of suppression are known: genotypic suppression in which a second mutation results in permanent alteration of the translation process; and phenotypic suppression in which added substances allow temporary nonheritable alterations in the interactions of translation components to occur.

Genotypic suppression

When the effects of a primary mutation are eliminated by a secondary mutation the latter is called a suppression mutation. Such suppressor mutations are classified as intragenic suppressors if they are located in the same gene as the original mutation; or extragenic suppressors if they are located in a different gene, or even a different chromosome, than the original mutation.

In intragenic suppression the secondary mutation is found in the same gene and cancels the deleterious effect of the primary mutation. Several examples can be cited: (1) a missense mutation followed by another missense mutation; (2) a frameshift mutation followed by another frameshift mutation of opposite sign; and (3) a nonsense codon which reverts not back to the original codon, but to another codon which allows a functional protein to be made.

Extragenic (or intergenic) suppression occurs when the suppressor is located on a gene other than the one containing the primary mutation. These suppressors must, therefore, influence the expression

Genetic suppression occurs when _____

_____

_____.

```
                    AMINO
                    ACID
            CODON   SIGNAL
            UGG  =  Tryptophan

Missense ↑      ↓  Nonsense

            UAG  =  Stop signal

Nonsense ↑      ↓  Missense

            UAU  =  Tyrosine
```

Genotypic/phenotypic suppression

occurs when a second mutation

"corrects" harmful effects of an

earlier mutation.

of the primary mutation by virtue of an alteration in a second functional unit of the translation process. The biochemical basis of the type of extragenic suppression that has been described in most detail involves synthesis of specific species of tRNA's.

Phenotypic Suppression

Streptomycin and other antibiotics belonging to the aminoglycoside family of antibiotics are known to cause "ambiguities" in amino acid incorporation; i.e., codon recognition of other amino acids at low frequencies. A translation error of this sort is sufficient to allow insertion of a proper, or at least compatible, amino acid at a position that is otherwise mutant. This sort of change results in a translation error which allows the synthesis of a small amount of active protein.

Examples of intragenic suppression

1. _____

   _____

2. _____

   _____

3. _____

   _____

Effects of Some Common Mutagens on DNA

Mutagen	Mechanism	Induced DNA Alteration
5-Bromouracil	Base analogue	T C transition
2-Aminopurine	Base analogue	A G transition
Nitrous acid	Base deamination	A G and C T transitions
Ethyl ethanesulfonate	Alkylation of quanine	Transition or transversion
Acridine dyes	Intercalation between bases	Frame-shift
Ultraviolet irradiation	Pyrimidine dimerization	Frame-shift, transversion CT transition, deletion
Ionizing Radiation	Free radical formed	Chromosomal strand breakage

GENE TRANSFER

Three types of gene transfer take place in bacteria. All involve a unidirectional transfer of genetic material from donor to recipient cells.

TRANSFORMATION

Transformation is the DNA-mediated transfer of a limited amount of genetic information from a disrupted to an intact cell. DNA is obtained from the donor cell either naturally by cell lysis, or artificially by a chemical extraction procedure, and is added to the recipient cells. Once DNA is taken up by the recipient cells, recombination of any marker can take place, and the cell is said to be transformed. Native double stranded DNA is the form most effective in transformation.

The Recipient

For successful transformation the recipient cells must be in a particular physiological state, called competence. The duration of the state is restricted to the late logarithmic phase of growth. Only competent cells can trap or bind the donor DNA to the recipient cells. Once the donor DNA is taken into the cell, integration of the donor DNA is accomplished by recombination. The DNA forms a partial diploid with the bacterial chromosome. When DNA replication occurs, 1 daughter will be a transformant.

Once donor DNA is taken into the competent recipient cell, integration occurs by _____.

Enzymes involved include

1. _____

2. _____

3. _____

(refer to "recombination" p. 45 for answer).

Gene transfer between bacteria is accomplished by 3 different processes:

1. _____

2. _____

3. _____.

Competence Factor is an extracellular protein that binds DNA to receptors on the cell; DNAse at cell surface degrades 1 strand and the other enters the cell.

4. _____

5. _____

TRANSDUCTION

Transduction is the type of gene transfer mediated by a bacteriophage, and involves the transfer of a limited amount of genetic information from a lysed donor cell to an intact recipient cell.

Generalized transduction occurs when a bacteriophage has the capacity to transfer any of the genes of the bacterial chromosome. Following infection of phage into bacteria, the virus particles multiply, making new enzymes, DNA, and coat protein (the assembly process is called encapsidation). Occasionally, a mistake is made during the assembly of the phage and a piece of bacterial DNA is packaged into the phage coat protein. This is the transducing particle, and since it contains little or no phage DNA, it cannot replicate further. Upon lysis of the bacteria, the phage particles are released, with the transducing particles making up only a small percentage of the total virus particles. A generalized transducing phage can pick up genes from any region of the bacterial chromosome.

Specialized transduction occurs when a particular phage strain can transduce only a few restricted genetic markers. These bacteriophages are temperate phages which during lysogeny integrate into a specific site on the bacterial chromosome. Upon induction of the prophage into the lytic cycle, genes adjacent to the prophage insertion point are occasionally carried along with the phage chromosome.

Abortive transduction occurs when the added piece of chromosome from a transducing phage fails to recombine or replicate, but still functions.

Gene transfer mediated by

bacteriophage is called

_____.

It is a generalized process if

_____

_____.

It is a specialized transfer if

_____

_____.

If the added DNA fails to replicate

the process is called

_____

_____.

49

BACTERIOPHAGES

Viruses that specifically infect bacteria are called bacteriophages, or simply phages. The life cycle of a virulent bacteriophage consists of infection, intracellular development and assembly into a complete phage, and lytic release of new progeny phage; this is called the lytic cycle. Bacteriophages called temperate phages can provoke one of two responses upon infection into a host cell; the lytic cycle (as above) or lysogeny. In lysogeny, the phage chromosome is integrated and replicates in concert with the host chromosome. The integrated phage chromosome is called a prophage, and the bacterial cell containing the prophage is called a lysogen. Lysogenic bacteria continue cell division indefinitely, and may lose the prophage in one of two ways; by the return of the prophage to the lytic cycle, or by spontaneous loss of the prophage. In the former case, bacteria are lysed and progeny phage are released, whereas in the latter case, bacteria retain their viability.

The Lytic Cycle

The lytic cycle of phage multiplication consists of the following steps:
1) absorption
2) penetration
3) intracellular development
4) maturation
5) lysis

1) <u>Absorption</u>. This process involves the presence of both an absorption organ on the phage and a highly specific receptor site on the bacteria. Phage resistance occurs if the host cell modifies its receptor molecule.

2) <u>Penetration</u>. The attachment of the tail fibers and pins to the cell surface triggers a contraction of the tail sheath. This results not only in the penetration of the tail core into the cell wall, but also a syringe-like action discharging the DNA into the host cell.

3) <u>Intracellular Development</u>. Intracellular development begins immediately after infection, with transcription of the phage DNA by host RNA polymerase. The phage mRNA is translated by the protein synthesizing machinery of the host and forms a number of new proteins called "early" proteins.

The next step is replication of nucleic acid. In dsDNA phages replication proceeds by the general mechanism of DNA synthesis. In ssDNA phages a complementary strand of DNA is synthesized (the dsDNA replicative form) which serves as a template for the synthesis of both mRNA and new phage DNA.

Shortly after replication begins, the "late" proteins begin to appear. Among the late proteins synthesized are subunits for phage components, as well as the enzyme lysozyme. This enzyme attacks the mucopeptide of the host cell wall and is primarily responsible for lysis and release of progeny phage.

4) **Assembly.** Once all the structural components are synthesized, maturation begins. The initial step involves the condensation of DNA, possibly with the aid of positively charged proteins, called internal proteins. The capsid subunits assemble around the condensed DNA to form the head. The tail and tail fibers are also formed independently and assemble to form the complete phage.

5) <u>Lysis</u>. The final step in phage multiplication is the lytic release of progeny phage. Lysis involved two or more gene products; at least one involved with an action on the membrane, and the other the action of lysozyme on the mucopeptide portion of the cell wall.

LYSOGENY

Definition

The stable (integrated) association of a temperate phage chromosome, in the prophage state, with the bacterial chromosome is called lysogeny. The prophage contains all the genetic information of the phage; however these genes are repressed.

Lysogen Formation

Following temperate phage infection, there is a critical period in which the viral particle either enters the lytic cycle or the lysogenic state. If lysogeny is to occur, this will be initiated by the synthesis of an mRNA which codes for a repressor protein. The repressor binds to the phage DNA in a region called the immunity region. This binding results in repression of virtually all phage directed syntheses and prevents the phage from entering the lytic cycle. The repressed phage chromosome becomes integrated in the host chromosome and remains in the lysogenic state.

Integration and Excision

The next step is the attachment of the phage chromosome to the bacterial DNA. The phage chromosome circularizes by joining single stranded cohesive ends, which are linked together by DNA ligase. Reciprocal recombination occurs between the phage and bacterial DNA's resulting in a linear integration of the phage chromosome. Excision occurs by a reversal of the steps of integration.

1 = A; see p. 49
2 = B

Phage Conversion

Lysogeny often results in the expression of new characteristics by the bacterial population. These may be due to
1) expression of phage genes, or
2) the induction of previously silent bacterial genes.

A medically significant phage conversion system involves the relationship of C. diphtheria exotoxin (tox+). The gene responsible for the production of the diphtheria toxin is located on the chromosome of phage beta.

Phage conversion involving toxin production occurs in several other organisms. For example, erythrogenic toxin, the toxin responsible for the rash of scarlet fever, is produced by lysogenic strains of Streptococcus pyogenes. In addition, types C and D toxins of Clostridium botulinum are produced following infection of specific phages.

A. transduction
B. lysogeny
C. both
D. neither

1. Integration of donor bacterial DNA into host (recipient) cell
2. Integration of phage DNA into host (recipient) cell

(Answers at left)

CONJUGATION

Conjugation is a process of genetic
exchange between two bacterial strains which
is dependent upon cell to cell contact.
It is the major means by which Gram negative
bacteria acquire multiple drug resistance.

In conjugation there are two mating types;
the male is the donor and contains an F (for
"fertility") factor, and is referred to as
F+; the female is the recipient and because
it lacks an F factor is referred to as an F-.
When strains of opposite mating type are
allowed to grow together for a short period
of time, and undergo conjugation, the F
factor of the male replicates, transferring
one of its copies to the female recipient.
The recipient cell is converted to an F+
cell, now being capable of serving as a
donor. Thus, as long as growth continues,
the conjugation process can continue in an
infectious manner.

The F factor is a circular piece of DNA of
molecular weight 50 X 10^6 and codes for
approximately 40-60 proteins. Certain clones
of F+ cells are capable of transferring
chromosomal genes with increased efficiency,
resulting in a high frequency of
recombination (Hfr). These cells are called
Hfr's and arise from F+ cells in which the F
factor becomes integrated into the bacterial
chromosome. The F factor DNA contains a
region of homology with the bacterial
chromosome and a recombination event takes
place between the two DNA's such that the F
factor is inserted linearly into the
bacterial chromosome.

F' formation

The integration of the F+ factor into the
chromosome to form an Hfr is a reversible
process. In some instances, the F factor
brings along with it some of the chromosomal
genes, and in this state is termed an F'.
The chromosomal genes incorporated into the
circular F factor are passed on during
conjugation. This process is called
sexduction and results

Cell contact is a prerequisite for

_____.

The Male/Female donor contains a

factor, called an _____ factor.

During genetic exchange this

factor replicates and one copy

is transferred to the Female/Male

recipient, which is then

converted to an _____ cell.

This is the primordial sex

change operation.

in a high frequency transfer of the F factor and linked chromosomal genes. The recipient cell in sexduction now possesses the same properties as the donor; i.e., it is F+ and contains the added genes attached to the F factor.

Physiology of Conjugation

Male strains have a small tubular appendage which forms a bridge between male and female strains. This appendage is called the F pilus and is synthesized under the control of F, with up to five pili per cell. The function of the F pilus is to form a specific attachment between the male and female that will allow conjugation to proceed. The pilus contracts bringing the cells into close contact to facilitate transfer of the F factor.

Cell-to-cell contact, which is essential for conjugation is accomplished via a specialized appendage called the _____

_____.

IDENTIFY THE CELLS BELOW (F-, Hfr, F' and F+)

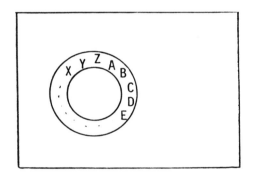

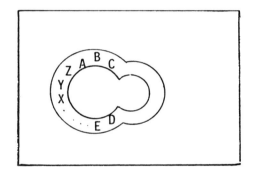

_____   _____

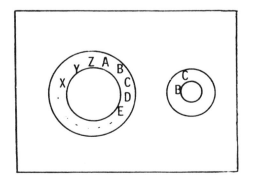

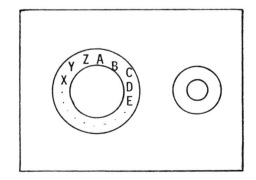

_____   _____

53

EXTRACHROMOSOMAL GENETIC ELEMENTS

Extrachromosomal genetic elements are often found in bacteria in addition to the normal chromosomal DNA. They are referred to as plasmids and are capable of autonomous replication in the cytoplasm. When an extrachromosomal element is capable of replicating either autonomously or integrated into the bacterial chromosome it is called an episome. Thus, the F factor which can alternatively exist as an F+ or an Hfr, is an example of an episome.

Phenotype functions mediated by plasmids include resistance to antibiotics, heavy metals, ultraviolet light, and specific phages, as well as production of antibiotics, bacteriocins, some toxins and other virulence enhancing factors (such as hemolysins, coagulase, etc.).

Bacteriocinogenic factors are extrachromosomal elements which produce bactericidal substances called bacteriocins. Bacteriocins differ from antibiotics in that they are proteins which act on only the same or closely related species of bacteria. Organisms which produce the bacteriocin are resistant to its action, whereas sensitive cells readily absorb the bacteriocin. Once absorbed, the bacteriocin initiates a highly specific action which leads to the death of the cell. This action differs for each type of bacteriocin, and may involve inhibition of oxidative phosphorylation, or cessation of DNA, RNA, or protein synthesis.

Resistance Transfer Factors

Resistance to antibiotics and other chemotherapeutic agents has been found to exist in a variety of microorganisms. In the Enterobacteriaceae, individual strains may show resistance to several antibiotics. Such multiple drug resistance is specified by an extrachromosomal element, called a resistance factor or R factor.

Plasmids which are capable of integration into the host genome are called

_____.

F factors are _____ or

_____ depending upon whether or not they have integrated into the host genome (answer below).

REVIEW STATEMENTS

For successful transformation the recipient cell must be in a particular physiologic state, called

_____.

The difference between generalized and specialized transduction is that in the former/latter the temperate bacteriophage integrates into the host genome at a specific site and, upon induction, genes adjacent to the prophage insertion site are carried along with the phage chromosome.

(answers = plasmids and episomes)

54

An R factor can be transferred by conjugation from one cell to another, and is often referred to as a resistance transfer factor (RTF). Genetic studies have shown that R factors consist of two distinct components, a transfer factor (RTF) and a resistance determinant (r determinant). The RTF is thought to be similar in function to an F factor, being responsible for both its own autonomous replication and conjugal transfer. The r determinant contains genes which specify resistance to various antibiotics. These two elements may exist independently, or associated together as an RTF:r determinant complex, i.e., R factor (perhaps similar to an F').

TRANSPOSONS - These are linear pieces of DNA, often containing r determinants, which promote their own transfer from 1 piece of DNA to another. For example, a transposon contained in the chromosome of a bacterium could transfer to a plasmid in the same cell; this complex may then be transferred to another bacteria by conjugation. The transposon might then dissociate itself from the plasmid and incorporate into the genome of the host cell. It can inactivate host genes during insertion.

The transposon has terminal repeating sequences of nucleotides on either side of the genes to be transferred which are mirror images of each other (they are palindromes). These are called INSERTION SEQUENCES which permit recognition of the correct area in the host genome, and insertion. The transposon has an endonuclease which will only "nick" DNA after a certain nucleotide sequence has occurred.

Transposon effects include mutations, and insertion of antibiotic resistance genes. Mutations can occur due to deletions or insertions, depending upon whether the transposon is coming or going.

Transposition occurs in the absence of recA function; therefore it is a type of _____ recombination (see p.45).

Two examples of episomes would be _____ and _____.

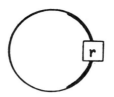 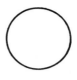

R factor   =   RTF   + r
                            determinant

TRANSPOSON

| I | GENES TO BE | S |
| S | TRANSFERRED e.g. r dtmt. | I |

Match the processes below with the components required for these processes to occur (answers on next page).

1. Sexduction   _____

2. Transduction   _____

3. Conjugation   _____

4. Transformation _____

COMPONENTS:
  A) Bacteriophage
  B) Cell-to-cell contact
  C) F' cell
  D) Competent cell
  E) Hfr cell
  F) F- cell
  G) F pilus
  H) Host bacterium

Which properties are common to

5. Plasmids and episomes?

6. Episomes and transposons?

  A) Autonomous replication
  B) Integration into host DNA
  C) Both
  D) Neither

55

RECOMBINANT DNA TECHNOLOGIES

The essential features in the construction and transfer of plasmid recombinant DNA molecules include: a method of specifically cleaving and then joining together DNA molecules from different sources; a source of carrier DNA capable of replicating itself and any foreign DNA joined to it; a method of transferring the composite DNA molecule to recipient bacterial cells; and finally, a method of detecting whether the recipient cells contain the recombinant DNA molecule.

Several specific enzymes are involved in the construction of plasmid recombinant DNA molecules. The first step involves a cleavage of a circular plasmid DNA molecule into a linear open form. One way of producing such a molecule is with E. coli R factor 1 restriction endonuclease (Eco R1), which makes staggered nicks in complementary strands of DNA at sites separated by several nucleotides. Different endonucleases recognize specific nucleotide sequences hence the DNA can be split at different sites. The resulting single-strand ends contain complementary sequences (cohesive ends) capable of hydrogen bonding again to form a circular molecule. Hydrogen bonding may also occur with single-strand regions of another plasmid or segment of foreign DNA cleaved by Eco R1 endonuclease. In this case, a recombinant DNA molecule is formed which is made up of the original plasmid and the segment of foreign DNA. The final step, sealing of the DNA molecules, is accomplished by DNA ligase, which catalyzes phosphodiester bonds to re-unite the DNA strands.

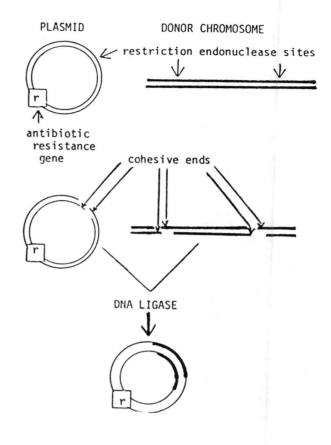

Answers to genetic transfer questions

1. B, C, E, F, G, H
2. A, H
3. B, F, G, H
4. D, H
5. A
6. B

Summary of essential features for gene cloning:

1. **Vector** - A source of carrier DNA; e.g., a **plasmid** or bacteriophage capable of gene transfer
2. **Connector** - A method of specifically splitting (**restriction endonuclease**) and rejoining (**DNA ligase**) DNA strands
3. **Selector** - A method of selecting the recombinant; e.g., **antibiotic resistance** gene carried on the vector
4. **Detector** - A method of detecting the product of the cloned (desired) gene; e.g., **ELISA** test for HBsAg

Barriers to expression of cloned eukaryotic genes in prokaryotic hosts include:

1. Promoters of eukaryotes are different; must supply prokaryote promoter.

2. Translation initiation signals (ribosome binding sites) of eukaryotes are different; must supply prokaryote binding sites.

3. Introns must be removed; most easily done by using cDNA.

How are these overcome?

1. RNA polymerase does not recognize the promoters of eukaryotic DNA. **The eukaryotic DNA segment is placed behind a prokaryotic promoter in the plasmid** which will allow RNA polymerase to attach and read the exon.

2. Ribosome binding sites are different in eukaryotic cells. This is overcome by **placing a prokaryotic ribosome binding site in front of the promoter in the plasmid**; this will provide a mechanism for efficient transcription and translation.

3. The eukaryotic DNA carries introns that must be removed. To avoid these we must start with mRNA. After the eukaryotic DNA is processed to mRNA we can "capture" the mRNA by using an affinity column coated with antibody to the desired protein. Alternately, an oligo(dT) column can be used to isolate mRNA with poly (A) tails. **Then utilizing reverse transcriptase, a sDNA can be produced. Using other DNA polymerase enzymes, dsDNA can then be produced.** This dsDNA codes for the mRNA without introns. This is called **cDNA** which stands for **complementary DNA.** The cDNA is then reinserted into a plasmid and is capable of being transfected into a cell and replicated.

Techniques that are employed in nucleic acid analysis

A. Polymerase chain reaction (PCR)

PCR is a method of **gene amplification** which produces a large amount of DNA in a short period of time. Requirements for this reaction include the following:

1. **Template DNA** containing the gene to be amplified.

2. **Oligonucleotides** spanning the region to be amplified.

3. **Taq polymerase** isolated from the thermophile*Thermus aquaticus*, which withstands elevated temperatures (70-95C) without denaturation.

4. **Thermal cycling chamber** to alternately denature DNA, renature it, and allow polymerization to occur.

The principle of the PCR is simple; with each temperature cycle there is a doubling of DNA strands.

At the lower temperature the DNA polymerase synthesizes complementary strands with the supplied oligonucleotides. The temperature is then raised to denature the dsDNA and separate the strands. The Taq enzyme withstands this elevated temperature and hence is still active when the chamber is cooled. It then synthesizes another set of dsDNA strands from the oligonucleotides provided. Thus one strand of DNA amplified over 15 cycles will produce 220,000 copies.

PCR has been useful for cloning specific genes, rapid identification of pathogens, and a variety of other uses. Procedures in which the PCR reaction can be utilized include:

1. For use in **amplifying DNA** present in small quantities so that it can be used to produce hormones, etc for human use. Many useful products have come out of this line of research, for example humulin (human erythropoietin), many monokines (IL-!), many cytokines (IL-2), etc.

2. To detect **HIV infection**
   It takes 1 month or more to mount an antibody response to the infection. With the use of PCR, one can detect the presence of HIV DNA in lymphocytes within 2-3 days post infection.

3. To **diagnose tuberculosis**
   With the use of PCR, one can detect as few as 10 tubercle bacilli in a sputum sample in a day or less.

B. Nucleic Acid hybridization

This technique is used to compare nucleic acids and to quantitate their concentration. It depends upon the ability of **complementary nucleic acid strands** to specifically **align and form stable double stranded associations.** The strand that is used as the detecting probe can be labeled with a fluorescent molecule, or it may be chemiluminescent, or radioactive thus its presence can be quantitated.

58

C.   **Restriction fragment length polymorphism analysis (RFLP)**

RFLP can be utilized to determined the relatedness of two samples of DNA or RNA. The procedure is performed as follows:

a.   Digest a piece of DNA from one source (via restriction endonucleases) and prepare a gel electrophoretic analysis; then digest and analyze DNA from a second source and compare their RFLP patterns to see if they are related.

b.   There are some **human diseases** we can specifically identify using RFLP.

   a.   In a number of **thalassemias**, we can detect them with RFLP.

   b.   RFLP can also be used to pick up **sickle cell anemias**.

   1.   In this disease, there is a normal hemoglobin called HBA and an abnormal hemoglobin called HbS.

   2,   HbS results from a glutamic acid to valine shift in amino acid position #6 which results from a single nucleotide change in the codon.

Utilization of Recombinant DNA Techniques in Gene Therapy

This has allowed us to take various kinds of retroviruses and use them to insert certain genes in target cells. If you take out the infectious genes of retroviruses, namely the **gag, pol** and **env** genes, the retrovirus becomes harmless in regard to changing or transforming cells of the host. These infectious genes are replaced with an innocuous gene and the virus becomes a **modified retrovirus**.

1.   If this modified retrovirus is placed in lymphocytes, you   can infect 1-10% of the cells and insert the desired gene.

2.   This approach has been used in gene therapy experiments in humans. The first experiment involved insertion of the gene for adenosine deaminase (ADA), the enzyme found lacking in those with ADA deficiency. Over 90% of the individuals with ADA deficiency also have a severe immune deficiency (SCID) .

3.   The experiment was performed by placing the ADA gene in a modified retrovirus, adding this retrovirus to T-lymphocytes removed from the patient, and then getting infection and recombination in the T-lymphocytes with inclusion of the ADA gene. The T lymphocytes are then reinjected into the individual who is found to have a functioning ADA gene and a relatively normal immune system.

4.   There are currently over 60 different protocols that are available for gene therapy. These include hypercholesterolemia, cystic fibrosis, and cancer.

REVIEW STATEMENTS

These should be used to strengthen and expand you understanding of Microbial Genetics. The statements are "factoids" that may help in the STEP 1 exam. You may wish to develop your own list to expand your knowledge base. If you have a spare sheet of paper available, white down the correct statement for every question you miss in going through review exams. This way you can avoid marking on the review exam (so you can use it again) and still have captured that fact for future review.

A **transversion** occurs when a purine in DNA is replaced by a pyrimidine.

Acridines cause frameshift mutants.

Restriction endonucleases break the chromosome at specific sites determined by nucleotide composition.

A secondary mutation which eliminates the effects of a primary mutation is a **suppressor**.

Mutations in the codon, the mRNA, the tRNA or the ribosome would all **effect translation**.

General recombination requires extensive DNA sequence homology.

UV light can cause **thymidine dimers**; repair enzymes can correct this error.

Polypeptide chain termination is caused by **nonsense** codons.

The bacteriophage-mediated transfer of genetic information from one bacteria to another is termed **transduction**.

Temperate bacteriophages can enter either the lytic cycle or the lysogenic state.

Bacteriophages are made of two molecular components, nucleic acid and protein.

DNA ligase is a phosphodiesterase.

Abortive transduction occurs in general transduction when the donated DNA fails to recombine or replicate, but still functions. A term that describes this event would be **complementation**.

Only **lysogenic** C. diphtheriae produce diphtheria toxin (are **toxigenic**).

The type of gene transfer mediated by purified DNA is **transformation**. **Competence** is a physiological state of recipient cells which is required for DNA binding in transformation.

Bacteriophage mediated transfer of genetic material is called **transduction**; a phage chromosome that has integrated into the bacterial DNA is a prophage.

Genetic complementation tests are used to determine whether two different different mutants carry mutations in the same cistron.

The conjugation bridge in bacteria is formed by **F pili**.

The **R-factor** of Gram negative enteric bacteria carries genes for **resistance** to several **antibiotics**.

Episomal transfer of resistance to antibiotics (RTF) occurs by the genetic mechanism called **conjugation**.

Following injection into a bacterial cell, the life cycle of a **virulent bacteriophage** consists of multiplication, packaging of nucleic acid, and cell lysis (release).

Following infection of sensitive bacteria by certain bacteriophages, the phage DNA becomes integrated in the host cell DNA and may influence or convert the recipient cell to produce new antigens or new toxins. A bacterium is said to be **lysogenic** when it contains a bacteriophage chromosome integrated into its own chromosome.

Genetic exchange between two bacterial strains which is dependent on cell to cell contact is **conjugation.**

The **polymerase chain reaction** requires a DNA polymerase, appropriate nucleotides for assembly, oligonucleotide primers and a DNA template. It is a technique used to replicate specific short regions of DNA exponentially in vitro.

Prokaryotic genes do not have intron sequences of noncoding DNA. prokaryotes can not splice out unnecessary sequences in mRNA hence **cDNA** is used to synthesize some mammalian proteins in bacteria.

The transfer of hereditary characteristics via cell-free DNA to competent recipient bacteria is termed **transformation; DNAse** interferes with this process.

A **generalized transducing particle** of *E. coli* containing host DNA can transfer any of the bacterial genes to a sensitive bacterial cell.

A mutation in DNA resulting in a **transition** results in one pyrimidine replacing another, it may be caused by the analog 5-bromouracil.

Excision repair involves the removal of thymidine dimers from ssDNA leaving a gap, and then utilizes the complementary strand as a template to resynthesize a new portion of DNA, which is sealed by **ligase.**

A **missense mutation** occurs when one base pair in a codon is replaced by another (with resultant replacement of one amino acid in the protein). **Nonsense codons** cause polypeptide chain termination due to a nucleotide change in the code which results in a **termination signal** (e.g., UGA).

Extrachromosomal, autonomously replicating circular DNA segments are called **plasmids.** Episomes are plasmids that have the ability to also replicate as a part of the cell's own DNA.

Recombination occurs due to breakage and reunion of chromosome strands.

For successful **transformation** the recipient cell must be in a particular physiologic state called **competence.**

Conjugation is a process of genetic exchange between two bacterial cells which is dependent upon cell-to-cell contact.

The F+ cell is the male "donor", F- female cells are the recipients, which are converted to F+ as a consequence of **conjugation.** In **Hfr** strains the F factor DNA integrates into the chromosome of the host cell. **F'** cells are those which have a piece of donor chromosome DNA that has been transferred along with the F factor.

Transposons are linear pieces of DNA, often containing **r determinants**, which promote their own transfer from one piece of DNA to another. Transposons encode a protein that catalyzes transposition (**transposase**). They are flanked by **insertion sequences**, which are the unique nucleotide sequences which permit recognition and insertion of the genes into the chromosome.

The enzyme that splits the plasmid chromosome for recombination is a **restriction endonuclease.** DNA annealing of the "new" DNA into the plasmid is accomplished by **DNA ligase.**

Bromouracil induces mutations through mispairing when it is incorporated into DNA as a structural analog of thymidine.

Alkylating agents such as nitrogen mustard and nitrosoguanidine react with guanine residues and cause improper base pairing during DNA replication.

Endonucleases do not digest DNA in the cell of origin because these cells have a **methylase** in the cytoplasm that methylates the DNA and protects it.

Restriction enzymes are of a group of bacterial **endonucleases** that cleave DNA at or near specific recognition sequences. The **Restriction fragment** is the piece of DNA produced by cleaving a larger fragment with a restriction enzyme

61

MICROBIAL GENETICS REVIEW EXAM

SELECT THE SINGLE BEST COMPLETION FOR EACH QUESTION BELOW.

1. The abnormal excision of a prophage and the incorporation of adjacent genes into a phage is one of the events leading to

   A. abortive tranduction.
   B. generalized transduction.
   C. specialized transduction.
   D. lysogenic conversion.
   E transposition.

2. Sequence specific enzymes that cleave DNA to give sticky ends are

   A. DNA methylases.
   B. DNA ligases.
   C. restriction endonucleases.
   D. beta-lactamases.
   E. photolyases.

3. The expression of prophage genes that confer a new phenotype to the bacteria, such as the production of diphtheria toxin, is termed

   A. prophage immunity.
   B. superinfection immunity.
   C. prophage induction.
   D. lysogeny.
   E. lysogenic conversion.

4. Conjugation

   A. is a mechanism of plasmid transfer.
   B. occurs only with temperate bacteriophages.
   C. can be inhibited by the addition of DNAse to the gene transfer mixture.
   D. requires the participation of a competent recipient.
   E. occurs optimally when both donor and recipient strains are F minus.

5. The addition of DNAse to a donor-recipient mixture will inhibit the following type of gene transfer:

   A. conjugation.
   B. transformation.
   C. transduction.
   D. transposition
   E. sexduction.

6. Specialized transduction

   A. transfers all genes of the chromosome with equal frequency.
   B. requires competent cells.
   C. is accomplished with phage particles obtained by induction of lysogens.
   D. is always accomplished with virulent bacteriophages.
   E. requires cell to cell contact of donor and recipient.

7. Plasmid mediated resistance to antibiotics may result in

   A. the formation of an altered peptidoglycan in the cell wall.
   B. the production of enzymes capable of inactivating the antibiotic.
   C. the induction of new antibiotic synthesis by the cell.
   D. production of nucleases to cleave antibiotic-producing transposons.
   E. altered ability of a cell to repair damage to DNA.

8. Transposable elements are capable of causing mutations in cells by

   A. the induction of thymidine dimers.
   B. direct insertion into a gene.
   C. the inhibition of SOS repair functions.
   D. combining specifically with DNA polymerase I.
   E. virtue of the fact that they possess a reverse transcriptase capable of synthesis of new DNA.

9. Thymidine dimers are formed in DNA due to the effect of

   A. ionizing radiation.
   B. ultraviolet radiation.
   C. alkylating gents.
   D. photoreactivation.

10. If DNA is damaged by an alkylating agent causing interstrand links, the most effective type of repair would be

    A. direct repair.
    B. photoreactivation.
    C. excision repair.
    D. post-replication repair.
    E. suppression.

11. A genetic element capable of moving from one chromosome to another that is independent of recA function is a

    A. transvertant.
    B. transformant.
    C. transposon.
    D. transuctant.
    E. transvestite.

12. A method of gene amplification which produces large amounts of DNA in a short period of time is

    A. specialized transduction.
    B. recombination.
    C. complementation.
    D. polymerase chain reaction.
    E. lysogenic conversion.

13. In clinical settings the acquisition of multiple antibiotic resistance by enteric Gram-negative bacteria most often involves

    A. conjugative plasmids.
    B. transducing phage.
    C. nonconjugative plasmids.
    D. spontaneous mutation.
    E. transformation of competent recipients.

14. Autonomously replicating DNA molecules that can serve as vehicles for DNA transfer are called

    A. selectors.
    B. bacteriogenic factors.
    C. connectors.
    D. vectors.

15. Restriction endonucleases are enzymes found in bacteria that

    A. degrade DNA sequentially beginning at the 5' end.
    B. cleave DNA at sequence-specific sites to yield either sticky (single stranded) or blunt ends.
    C. form phophodiester bonds at the site of a single strand break in DNA.
    D. are an integral part of genetic recombination.
    E. cleave a portion of the gene that is transcribed but do not appear in the final mRNA transcript.

16. Eukaryotic DNA contains introns that present a barrier to successful transcription in prokaryotic organisms. To overcome this obstacle, we can employ what additonal reagent?

    A. ECOR1 endonuclease.
    B. bacteriocinogenic factor.
    C. cDNA.
    D. intron-recognizing primer oligonucleotides.
    E. intron-specific endonucleases.

17. Which of the following is **NOT** true of transposons?

    A. They are genetic units that move within and between different DNA molecules.
    B. They require RecA for homologous recombination.
    C. They are flanked by inverted repeat regions of DNA at their ends.
    D. They may cause mutations by insertion into a gene.
    E. They may contain genes which encode antibiotic resistance.

18. Restriction endonucleases recognize specific nucleotide sequences and may do all of the following **EXCEPT**

    A. methylate the sequence so it can't be   cleaved.
    B. cleave the sequence to give sticky (cohesive) end.
    C. cleave the sequence to give flush (blunt) end molecules.
    D. join the nucleotide chains to effect repair.

19. Point mutations and base pair substitutions are caused by all of the following **EXCEPT**

    A. alkylating agents.
    B. nitrous acid.
    C. pyrimidine analogs.
    D. acridines.
    E. sulfur mustards.

20. Bacteria are able to exchange genetic information by all of the following methods **EXCEPT**

    A. conjugation.
    B. transformation.
    C. transposon insetion.
    D. transduction.
    E. complementation.

21. All of the following are genetic processes which enable cells to overcome a mutation **EXCEPT**

    A. repair.
    B. recombination.
    C. suppression.
    D. complementation.
    E. lysogeny.

22. DNA vectors used in DNA technology should have all of the following properties **EXCEPT**

    A. a selectable phenotype.
    B. single sites for restriction enzymes.
    C. autonomous replication.
    D. ability to transfer genes to viable cells.
    E. intervening sesequences.

23. Bacteria are simple genetic units with all of the following properties **EXCEPT**

    A. they are haploid.
    B. their genetic material is organized into a single circular chromosome.
    C. they use the same genetic code as eukaryotic cells.
    D. their introns are highly conserved genetic repeats.
    E. their genotypes and phenotypes are the same

24. All of the following are true of recombinant DNA technology **EXCEPT**

    A. utilizes enzymes such as restriction endonuclease.
    B. allows the combining of prokaryotic and eukaryotic DNA in the same organism.
    C. has the potential of cloning any single gene.
    D   can utilize DNA as a donor gene.
    E. requires a heat labile DNA polymerase.

25. Mechanisms of plasmid specified antibiotic resistance include all of the following **EXCEPT**

    A.   detoxification, or alteration of the antibiotic to an inactive state.

    B.   interference with transport of the antibiotic into the cell.

    C.   alteration of the target site such that it no longer interacts with the antibiotic.

    D.   misreading of the genetic code by the antibiotic to insert missense amino acids in the protein.

26. Polymerase chain reaction techniques now make it possible to do all of the following **EXCEPT**

    A.   synthesize viral vaccine components

    B.   identify pathogens with specific probes

    C.   synthesize human hormone

    D.   prove identity of different DNA samples.

27. All of the following are true of recombinant DNA technology **EXCEPT**

    A.   is possible because of the utilization of enzymes such as restriction endonucleases, DNA polymerase, and DNA ligase.

    B.   allows the combining of prokaryotic and eukaryotic DNA in the same organism.

    C.   has the potential of cloning any single gene.

    D.   can not use cDNA as a primer.

28. All of the following are ingredients of the polymerase chain reaction **EXCEPT**

    A.   thermal cycling chamber.

    B.   Taq polymerase.

    C.   oligonucleotides spanning the region to be amplified.

    D.   template DNA containing the gene to be amplified.

    E.   plasmids with antibiotic resistance genes.

Directions (items 29-32) Match each statement describing a characteristic of genetic exchange with the transfer mechanism or mechanisms that demonstrate that feature. **AN ANSWER MAY BE USED MORE THAN ONCE, OR NOT AT ALL.**

A.	Transformation	E.	Education
B.	Transduction	F.	Complementation
C.	Conjugation	G.	Suppression
D.	Mutation	H.	Insertional inactivation

29. This process is sensitive to the presence of DNAse in the suspension medium

30. This process requires that the bacteria be in a state of competence

31. This process involves packaging and transfer of DNA by a bacteriophage

32. This process is the most common means whereby bacteria become resistant to antibiotics

KEY

1.	C	6.	C	11.	C	16.	C	21.	E	26.	D
2.	C	7.	B	12.	D	17.	B	22.	E	27.	D
3.	E	8.	B	13.	A	18.	D	23.	D	28.	E
4.	A	9.	B	14.	D	19.	D	24.	E	29.	A
5.	B	10.	D	15.	B	20.	B	25.	D	30.	A
										31.	B
										32.	C

REVIEW OF

IMMUNOLOGY

This first portion of this section will deal with Basic Immunology (innate immunity, complement, the immune response and serologic reactions). The second section contains a review of clinical aspects of immunology (hypersensitivities, autoimmunity, immune deficiency tumor immunity and transplantation immunology).

INNATE IMMUNITY

Immunity (resistance to, or assistance with, an infectious disease) can be acquired by various means which are summarized below.

Role of

Recipient	Method	Examples	Duration*
Passive	Natural	IgG across placenta IgA in colostrum**	months days
	Artificial	Horse antitoxin Human gamma globulin	days weeks
Active	Natural	Recovery from infection —clinical or subclinical	months to years
	Artificial	Vaccination with agent*** or product	months to years

*duration of immunity will vary with:
1. Amount and class of gamma globulin
2. Foreignness of gamma globulin
3. Nature of infectious agent (i.e., there is no post-infection immunity with some agents; e.g., Staphylococcus), and
4. Type of vaccine (attenuated are better than killed)

** gut immunity only; sIgA does not get into the circulation.

***stimulates production of specific, protective antibody which enhances phagocytosis, neutralizes the toxin, etc, dependent upon the nature and composition of the vaccine.

The immunoglobulin which crosses the human placental barrier is _____.

Transplacental immunity lasts 4 - 6 (days/weeks/months/years) in humans.

Recovery from measles should induce an _____ immunity which will persist for (days/weeks/months/years).

Secretory IgA in colostrum is a(an) _____ immunity. It is effective in protecting the gut/CNS).

Human gamma globulin will provide a passive immunity of longer/shorter duration than would horse antitoxin.

The major phagocytic cells of the body are the _____ and the _____. (see next page for the answer)

The external body surfaces form the first line of defense. These include the skin and epithelium lining the alimentary and respiratory tracts. This barrier is also bathed in secretions which contain antimicrobial substances like lysozyme. Most secretions have a flushing action as well which helps rid the body of microbes.

CELLULAR DEFENSE MECHANISMS

1. Principal cells are polymorphonuclear leukocytes (PMN's) and monocytes in the blood, and tissue macrophages. While these are not the only cells which phagocytize, they are most important.
   A. All are capable of ameboid movement; that is, they can move in and out of blood vessels.
   B. Chemotaxis - they move because they are attracted by certain chemicals, i.e. tissue components and complement component C5a, as well as leukotriene B4 and endotoxin (LPS).
   C. Once close enough to the target, they engulf it.
   D. They digest, or attempt to digest, particles engulfed.

2. Natural Killer (NK) cells are lymphocytes which are present prior to antigen stimulation; their numbers do not increase with immunization. They react with foreign tissues, tumors and virus-infected cells and rid the body of them. They are neither T nor B cells, but have some membrane markers of each. They also have a monocyte marker.

3. Phagocytosis - First a phagosome is formed by the phagocyte when it engulfs the particle and surrounds it with a part of its cell membrane. This pinches off and moves into the cell cytoplasm. In the cytoplasm are lysosomes, or membrane-bound bags of proteolytic enzymes, which fuse with the phagosome (phagolysosome). Phagocytosis is accompanied by an increase in lactic acid production, O_2 uptake and hexose monophosphate shunt (HMP) activity.

4. Opsonization - Certain factors increase the efficiency of phagocytosis. Surfaces, such as the vascular wall and fibrin clots, provide a support upon which the phagocytic cell operates. Antibody and complement opsonize by reacting with Fc and C3b receptors in the phagocytic cell membrane. In addition, certain microbial products, such as endotoxin, increase the efficiency of the reticuloendothelial system (RES).

The essential steps in phagocytosis include:

1. _____

2. _____

3. _____

Chemotactic factors which are generated during complement activation include _____ and _____.

The energy required for efficient phagocytosis is generated by the _____.

Opsonization, the facilitation of the engulfment process, is enhanced by

1. the Fc portion of the antibody.

2. C3b molecules that adhere to the surface of the particle.

3. Both

4. Neither

(Answer on next page)

5. Killing occurs via the contents of the lysosomes, which include:

A. Myeloperoxidase + H_2O_2 + Halide (Cl or I): kills via halogenation of the organism, also toxic hypochlorite is generated, as are toxic aldehydes. H_2O_2, singlet oxygen, superoxide anion and hydroxyl ion) also come from the HMP shunt.

B. Lysozyme is another antimicrobic found in lysosomes, as well as in tears, saliva, and most body fluids. This enzyme attacks the cell wall and lyses it, both in Gram+ and − bacteria. It is a mucopeptidase.

C. Fatty Acids − are antimicrobial.

D. Toxic Proteins − basic proteins are found in lysosomes. They are very effective antimicrobial agents and seem to be simple polypeptides, as (Arg)n and (Lys)n.

E. Phagocytin − kills microorganisms and is more active at low pH.

F. Acid Hydrolases − phosphatases, glucuronidase, cathepsin, etc.

6. Cellular defense mechanisms are also enhanced by substances released from monocytes (monokines) which effect other aspects of resistance.

A. Interleukin I is a major product which activates many other cells of the body and also is active in fever (it is endogenous pyrogen).

B. Prostaglandins which increase vascular permeability

C. Tumor necrosis factor

D. Interferon alpha

Antimicrobial contents of the lysosome include:

1. lactoferrin, an Fe binding protein plus

2. _____

3. _____

4. _____

5. _____

6. _____

7. _____

_____ kills bacteria by

halogenation of essential microbial

components such as transport proteins.

The mucopeptidase which destroys the

peptidoglycan component of the cell

wall is _____.

(Answer = 3)

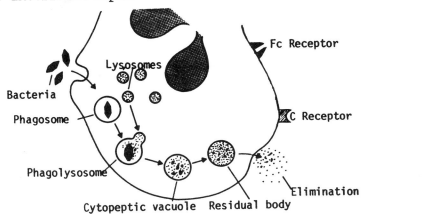

Bacteria
Lysosomes
Fc Receptor
Phagosome
C Receptor
Phagolysosome
Cytopeptic vacuole   Residual body
Elimination

69

COMPLEMENT

The complement system is made up of 9 serum proteins (complement components) and several regulatory factors which control the interactions of the complement components. The divalent cations Ca++ and Mg++ are also involved in function of the complement system. Macrophages produce many C proteins.

Many of the complement components are produced in _____.

FUNCTIONS OF COMPLEMENT

1. <u>Immune cytolysis</u>. This is the antibody and complement mediated destruction of cell membrane integrity.

2. <u>Acceleration of acute inflammation</u>. When complement reacts with antigen-antibody complexes or sensitized cells, peptides are enzymatically split from some of the complement components. These peptides accelerate acute inflammation in several ways. One of these (C5a) enhances the migration of polymorphonuclear leukocytes, thus it is called a chemotactic factor. C3b causes opsonization (allowing cells which have the innate ability to phagocytize to do so more efficiently). C3a and C5a are also called anaphylatoxins and cause mast cells to release histamine. In turn, histamine alters vascular permeability and smooth muscle tone.

3. <u>Immune adherence</u>. Membranes bearing certain activated complement components, e.g. C3b, behave as though they were sticky. This phenomenon may be important <u>in vivo</u> in aggregation of bacteria, leukocytes, platelets, etc. and play a role in complement acceleration of blood clotting and phagocytosis.

Functions of complement include:

1. _____

2. _____

3. _____

4. _____

5. _____

6. _____

SUMMARY OF COMPLEMENT'S SEQUENTIAL REACTION CASCADE

E + A $\longrightarrow$ EA + C1 $\longrightarrow$ EAC1 + C4, C2 $\longrightarrow$ EAC14b2b + C3 $\longrightarrow$ EAC14b2b3b

$+$

C5, C6, C7

$\downarrow$

(LYSIS) $\longleftarrow$ EAC14b2b3b5b6789 $\longleftarrow$ $\longleftarrow$ C8, C9 $+$ EAC14b2b3b5b67

70

COMPLEMENT NOMENCLATURE

The complement components are distinct serum proteins, all of which acting together have the cytolytic activity of complement. Other proteins are involved with complement as regulators, activators, inactivators, etc.

Classically, EA is used to designate the immune complex; E is the antigen (erythrocyte in the original work) and A is the antibody. The C components bind to EA to form a very large macromolecular complex, written EAC142356789. The numbers indicate the order in which components bind to the complex. As complement components are activated, they may bind to a growing complex or in the immediate vicinity of the sensitizing antibody.

MECHANISMS OF COMPLEMENT SYSTEM ACTIVATION

THE CLASSICAL PATHWAY

When IgM or IgG (except IgG-4) antibody reacts with an antigen, there is a rearrangement in the structure of the Fc portion of the antibody, forming a C1 binding site in the CH2 domain.

C1 is a complex macromolecule made up of 3 polypeptides. The C1 molecule contains a calcium ion (necessary for activity) and 3 polypeptides C1q, C1r, and C1s. C1q is the peptide which binds to the modified Fc portion of an immune complex. Binding of the C1q causes a change in the structure of the C1q which in turn leads to rearrangement of structure in the C1r and C1s peptides. The C1s peptide acquires an enzymatic activity as a result of this arrangement. Activated C1s becomes a <u>serine</u> <u>esterase</u>. Under physiological conditions, C1q, C1r, and C1s are always bound to each other and to Ca^{++}.

Match the following: (see previous page)

1. Anaphylotoxins

2. Chemotactic factor

3. Opsonin

4. Immune adherence

5. Histamine release

    A. C1a
    B. C3b
    C. C3a
    D. C5a
    E. C5b67

The most efficient immunoglobulin

at activating complement is _____.

THE INITIAL EVENT IN THE COMPLEMENT-MEDIATED LYSIS OF A CELL MEMBRANE

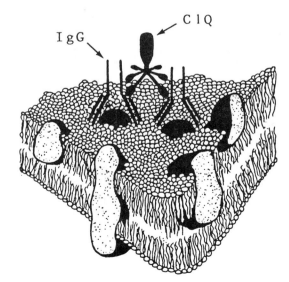

71

EAC1 is the first complex containing an activated complement component. C1 esterase (C1a) converts native C4 and C2 into activated states. Activated C4 binds to EAC1 to form EAC14b. Activated C4 binds to receptor sites on membranes, usually (but not necessarily) the same membrane to which the C1 is bound. C2 binds to activated C4 forming EAC14b2b. The C2b portion of this complex is enzymatically active. C4b2b has the descriptive name "C3 convertase."

Through the action of C3 convertase, C3 is split into active peptides. One of these, C3b, binds to the membrane forming EAC14b2b3b.

The C3 fragments formed in the classical pathway are listed below. C3a and C3b may also be produced from C3 by other proteolytic enzymes (e.g., trypsin, plasmin, Hageman factor, etc.).

1. Opsonic factor (C3b) - Associated with increased activity of polymorphonuclear leukocytes; when membranes are opsonized they are more susceptible to the phago cytic activity of PMN.
2. Anaphylotoxins (C3a and C5a) Cause mast cells and basophils to release their histamine (histamine in turn causes increased capillary permeability and vasodilitation). C5a also attracts polymorphonuclear leukocytes (chemotaxis).

Those complexes containing both C3 convertase and C3b activate C5, 6 and 7. C5 is split into fragments, C5a and C5b; C5b binds to C6 and C7 forming C5b67 which is also bound to membranes. These steps also lead to the formation of a biologically active factor, C5a or anaphylotoxin II, which also is a chemotactic factor.

C8 then adds to the growing complex to form membrane bound C5b678, and slow dissolution of the membrane begins. (This is the effector step in the "attack sequence" of the complement cascade). The rate of membrane des-truction is enhanced by the addition of C9 to form the completed complex.

The biologically active components

of the Complement cascade are:

Anaphylotoxins

    1._____

    2._____

Chemotaxin

    1._____

Opsonin

    1._____

Membrane attack complex

    1._____

Regulators of Complement activation
include; C1 esterase inhibitor
          C3b inactivator (factor I)
          Decay accelerating factor (DAF)
          Factor H
          C4b bindng protein
These proteins interfere with complement component activation and/or destabilize the amplification complexes.

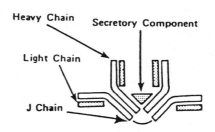

Secretory IgA Globulin (sIgA)

The antibody molecule above does/does not activate C by the classic pathway.

THE ALTERNATE PATHWAY (PROPERDIN PATHWAY)

The alternate (non-antibody dependent) pathway of complement activation involves three additional serum proteins, factor B, factor D and Properdin. C3 undergoes a natural decay process in the body and C3b is produced at a low level. This is usually inactivated by complexing with Factor H (beta 1 H globulin) and C3b inactivator protein. If the C3b is bound to a protective surface such as a bacterial cell, LPS, zymosan, complex CHO's, or certain immune complexes then inactivation does not occur and the complement cascade distal to the C142 participation steps ensues. Bound C3b, in the presence of factor D and Mg++, cleaves factor B releasing a small peptide (Ba) and forming the alternate pathway C3 convertase, C3bBb. Properdin stabilizes the C3 convertase, forming C3bBbP which then is able to cleave C3 and C5 and complete the cascade to the membrane attack complex, C5b6789.

CLINICAL IMPLICATIONS

1. With the addition of C1 to form EAC1a, an alternate pathway with decay of the complex to form EA + free C1a may occur. The free C1a is enzymatically active, and it may cause trouble. Free C1a can activate subsequent components, and if it does this in a fluid phase (as opposed to a membrane-bound phase), symptoms of systemic vasodilitation and inflammation occur. This is normally prevented by a protein that inhibits C1a called C1 esterase inhibitor. C1 esterase inhibitor slows generation of free C1a and blocks its enzymatic activity competitively. Hereditary angioneurotic edema (HAE) is a disease in which occasional spontaneous edema occurs. These individuals have a deficiency in C1 esterase inhibitor.
2. Hereditary deficiency of certain complement components is associated with recurrent bacterial infections. The most severe forms are the deficiencies of those components which are involved in opsonization and chemotaxis (C3 and C5). Absence of early C proteins is associated with an SLE-like disease.

C3b + B + C3bina = inactive C3b

+

AC (activating surface)

+

B

$\downarrow$ D, Mg++ cofactors

AC–C3bBb (C3 convertase)

+

P (properdin)

$\downarrow$

AC–C3bBbP (stabilized complex)

+

C567, C89

$\downarrow$

LYSIS

Congenital absence of C1 esterase inhibitor results in _____

_____

_____.

3. A protein has been discovered in the serum of patients with chronic membrano-proliferative glomerulonephritis which is able to stabilize the C3bBb:C3 convertase complex in a manner similar to that of Properdin. It has been suggested that this factor, called C3 nephritic factor (C3NeF), is an IgG immunoglobulin that is directed against a component of the C3bBb complex. This may explain the continuous alternate C pathway activation that accompanies this disease.

Complement levels are often decreased an autoimmune diseases and occasionally in acute infectious diseases. These changes are due to C utilization. A serious C consumption can occur during septic disease and is associated with disseminated intravascular coagulopathy.

5. Inherited deficiencies of certain complement components have been assoc-iated with increased incidence of infectious diseases. The deficiencies are usually those involving C components from C3 through the final membrane attack molecule, C9. Deficiencies of C5-9 have been associated with Gram negative coccal infections such as meningococcemia.

Complement Fixation Test
1. Useful in diagnosis of viral infections and syphilis
2. Comprised of 2 stages
   a. Test system
      Patient's serum
       +
      Known Antigen
       +
      Complement

   b. Indicator system
      Sheep RBCs
       +
      Hemolysin

3. If C is "fixed" (consumed) in 2a due to the Ag:Ab complexes, then there will be no lysis when step 2b is performed, i.e., a positive test.

There are several reasons why complement levels may be depressed, including such 4. things as

_____,

_____,

_____, and

_____.

If the complement is "fixed", the ery-

throcytes will/will not lyse; this means

there was/was not an antigen:antibody

reaction in the test system.

74

ANTIBODY STRUCTURE
AND FUNCTION

Antibodies are divided into 5 classes on
the basis of their antigenically distinct
heavy chains. Any one antibody molecule
will have 2 identical heavy chains per
unit. There are two types of light chains
called kappa and lambda, but in any one
antibody molecule the light chains are
both of the same type. There are subtle
differences in the constant region of the
heavy chains and light chains which are
called allotypes, and they are analogous
to the differences in blood type, i.e.,
they impart unique antigenic specificity
to the molecule. The allotypes are
designated Gm for gamma chain, Am for
alpha chain, and Km for kappa chain.
Heavy chain class is controlled by
isotypic determinants also found in the
constant region. Unique determinant
groups are found in the variable region,
associated with the antigen-binding (Fab)
capability of the molecule. These are
called idiotypes. Anti-idiotype Ab will
resemble the original antigenic determinant group.

Antigen binding occurs at the

variable/constant portion of the H/L/both

chain(s).

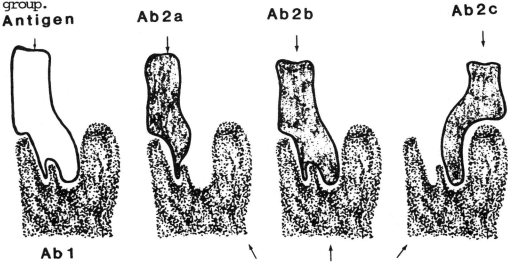

Ab 1 as Antigen

In the illustration above the antibody 1 idiotype, acting as an immunogen itself,
has induced the production of 3 different anti-idiotypic antibodies, Ab2a, Ab2b,
and Ab2c. Only one of these, Ab2b, is a perfect match and is immunologically
identical to the epitope which induced antibody 1.

Figure 1 is the structure of the IgG molecule, and this structure is also the same basic structure for all five classes. The molecule is composed of four polypeptide chains: two heavy and two light chains joined by disulfide bonds. Enzymatic treatment of this molecule with papain splits it into three fragments. The parts containing the heavy and ilght chains are called fragment antigen binding, or Fab, and this end of the molecule is the one that binds to the antigen. Each Fab molecule has a valence of 1. Pepsin splits below the disulfide interchain bond, producing a divalent molecule, $F(ab')_2$.

The fragment containing only heavy chains is called fragment crytstallizing, or Fc, and this portion binds serum complement, contains some carbohydrate, and is the constant region of the molecule. Fd refers to the heavy chain component of Fab. Since the immunoglobulin is a polypeptide, there must be a N terminal end and a C terminal end. The N terminus binds to the antigen while the C terminus dictates whether or not the molecule will pass through the placenta, fix complement, attach to mast cells, etc.

The variable and constant regions of each chain are divided into domains, which are compact, globular loops of the polypeptide stablized by S-S bonds. The light chains have 2 domains, V, and C, gamma and alpha chains have 4, mu and epsilon, 5.

Papain treatment of an immunoglobulin molecule splits it into the following fragments:

_____ and

_____ .

The Fc portion of the immunoglobulin molecule has several biological functions and/or chemical characteristics, among which are

_____ ,

_____ ,

_____ ,

_____ , and

_____ .

Figure 1. Component parts of an immunoglobulin G molecule.

FUNCTIONS

IgG is the only immunoglobulin that can cross the placenta. It has gamma heavy chains, is the most abundant antibody in serum and has the longest half life.

IgA is a variable molecule because it can exist as a monomer, a dimer or other polymeric forms. H chains are α type. A type of IgA is called secretory IgA, which is two IgA molecules joined together by a secretory component which enables the molecules to leave the secretory epithelial cell. The "J" or joining chain also aids in stabilizing the dimer. This antibody is responsible for the mucosal immunity involving·such secretions as saliva, colostrum and tears. It also helps protect the bronchial, intestinal and urinary tracts. It blocks adherence of pathogens to tissues and may also opsonize invading microbes.

IgM is a macroglobulin that exists as a monomer in B cell membranes and as a pentamer in serum, held together by S-S bonds and a single J chain. Its heavy chains are mu type. IgM is the most efficient Ab in C-mediated lytic reactions because only 1 molecule is needed to activate the cascade. It is the 1st antibody synthesized by a B cell and is also the major fetal antibody synthesized _in utero_. Elevated IgM levels in cord blood signify fetal infection.

IgD may constitute a primitive antigen receptor on lymphoid cells. It occurs on fetal and leukemic lymphocytes. Heavy chains are delta type.

IgE is responsible for the immediate types of hypersensitivity (atopy and anaphylaxis). It is involved in allergies such as asthma, hay fever and reactions to foods, as well as in parasitic infections. It appears to be involved in immunity to certain parasitic disease, e.g., ascariasis. Epsilon heavy chains are found in IgE. The molecule has a high affinity for mast cells and basophils.

	IgG Subclass			
	1	2	3	4
% of IgG	70	20	7	3
C binding	+	+	3+	0
Opsonizing	3+	+	3+	+

The Ig class switch occurs in a committed Ig-secreting cells. It is accompanied by a change in the constant heavy gene (change from CHmu to CHgamma). There is no change in the variable domain genes.

The blocking antibodies induced in atopic allergies are IgG.

How many **different** polypeptides are there in IgG _____

sIgA _____

IgM _____

77

IMMUNE RESPONSE

TERMS TO KNOW

<u>Thymus</u> <u>dependent</u> <u>areas</u> of lymph node –
Juxtamedullary (paracortical) areas
involved in cell mediated immunity.

<u>Thymus</u> <u>independent</u> <u>areas</u> – germinal
centers and medullary plasma cells
involved in antibody synthesis.

<u>Primary</u> <u>immune</u> <u>response</u> – first exposure
to Ag – mainly IgM Ab produced.

<u>Secondary</u> <u>immune</u> <u>response</u> – second expo-
sure – mainly IgG

<u>Booster</u> – anamnesis or memory, much more
rapid rise in Aby level

<u>Adjuvant</u> – substance which greatly
enhance the immune response

ANAMNESIS

The first response to antigen is mainly
IgM; there is a feedback to IgM and its
production is shut down. The cell then
switches to production of IgG. With the
booster antigen challenge, antibody goes
to a higher level and stays there longer.
The challenge boosts antibody production.
Immune memory depends on both B and T
cells, although T cells seem to be most
important. It takes far less Ag to
produce an anamnestic response than to
initially immunize.

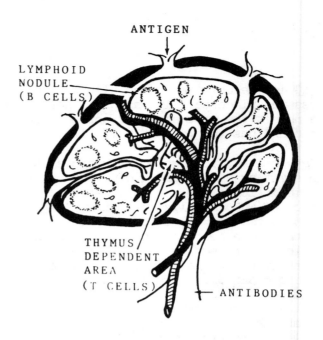

SIZE

+

IMMUNOGENICITY =   FOREIGNNESS

+

CHEMICAL COMPLEXITY

PHASES OF THE IMMUNE RESPONSE

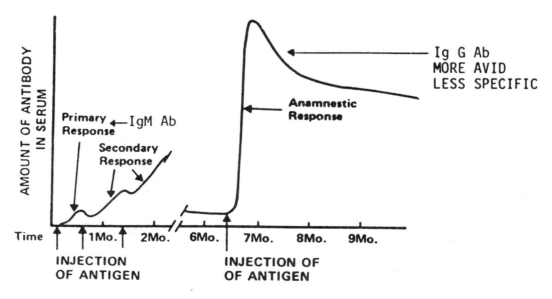

78

THE CELLULAR EVENTS OF THE IMMUNE RESPONSE

When an antigen enters a node (or the spleen), it first encounters a macrophage. It is processed and presented on the cell membrane. A lymphocyte with a membrane-bound IgM homologous to the antigen then reacts. The macrophage releases a mono-kine, Interleukin I, which stimulates the lymphocyte to divide and differentiate. In most immune responses there are 2 lymphocytes; a T helper cell, and a B cell (the plasma cell precursor). The T helper cell releases a lymphokine called Inter-leukin II which aids in the T cell proliferation. Other lymphokines are produced which aid in maturation, immuno-globulin classswitching, etc.

The interaction between the T and B lymphocytes is called collaboration. Both humoral and cellular immunities are produced to some degree, depending on the antigen and how it is administered.

Most immune responses are T dependent: all cell-mediated responses are, and most of the humoral ones also require a T helper cell. The few that do not are called T INdependent responses. The anti-gens which are responsible (T independent antigens) are usually composed of mono tonously repeating units (e.g., CHO, LPS). The responses are IgM in nature and do not have an anamnestic response. Some T inde pendent antigens are polyclonal B cell activators.

Macrophages are essential for immune responses. However, they do not produce antibody and, in contrast to B and T cells, do not demonstrate any selectivity in the antigens with which they react. Maturation of B and T cells is antigen independent; the antigen serves as a trigger to proliferation once the cell has become immunologically committed.

Stem cells arise in the bone marrow. Some mature there and become functional B cells which seed the peripheral lymphoid organs such as the spleen and nodes. Other stem cells migrate to the thymus where, under the influence of hormones such as thymosin produced by epithelial cells, they differentiate into mature T cells. Self reactive T cells are destroyed while developing in the thymus.

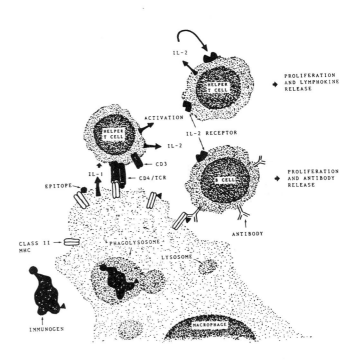

CELL INTERACTIONS IN HUMORAL IMMUNITY

The events which occur in the cellular collaboration depicted above are detailed in the left hand column. There are several lymphokines involved as enhancers of proliferation (see page 99); only 2 are shown here, Interleukins 1 and 2. Epitope presentation with the class II Major Histocompatibility Complex molecule is discussed in more detail on page 97. The helper T cell bears a molecule, CD4, which, in conjunction with the epitope-specific T cell receptor, (see CD4/TCR above) and the CD3 molecule, interacts with the "processed" epitope and initiates the activation process. An immunologically committed B cell, with monomeric IgM in its membrane, reacts with a homologous macrophage presented epitope and, under the influence of IL-2 and other lymphokines, begins the process of proliferation and differentiation which will culminate antibody synthesis and secretion by mature plasma cells.

IgM is the first immunoglobulin to be produced by the fetus (ca. 3 months). Cytoplasmic IgM is the first antibody to be seen; later it will also appear on the B cell membrane, and eventually, it will be secreted. IgG is the major immunoglobulin in fetal serum, due to the large amount which is acquired via the placenta (IgG of maternal allotype). Maternal IgG in newborn prevents optimal priming immediately after birth for the corresponding antigen. Elevated levels of IgM in cord blood may signify congenital infection (e.g., rubella or syphilis). IgA is not produced in utero: production beginning shortly after birth. Adult levels of these immunoglobulins are attained at approximately 1, 4 and 8 years, respectively. Adult IgE levels are not seen until 14-16 years of age. Both IgM and IgD are found on lymphocyte membranes in utero.

Haptens - These materials cannot induce antibody formation unless conjugated to a material which increases their size and the density of haptenic groups per molecule (e.g., carrier molecules). They will, however, react with the antibody induced, even in the absence of a carrier molecule. Most substances used to impart immunogenicity to haptens are antigenic themselves; in fact, in certain systems, they must be immunogenic to the recipient. The antibody induced to the hapten- carrier complex will be heterogenous; i.e., antibody vs. carrier, antibody vs. hapten and perhaps antibody vs. area of conjugation. The carrier effect demonstrates the importance of the carrier molecule in the anamnestic response to the hapten. A secondary response to the hapten will not occur if the carrier used in the booster injection is different from that employed to prime the animal.

Congenital infections will cause an increase in fetal IgG/IgM levels in cord blood.

> The null period is the time of greatest risk for an infant. It is when the maternal Ab is waning and the infant is just beginning to synthesis its own IgG.

Adult levels of most of the immunoglobulins are reached by the age of _____ years.

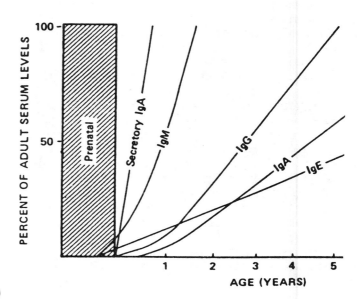

However, if the animal was immunized to the second carrier (without attached hapten) previously, then a normal anamnestic response to the hapten will occur. Thus priming in both the B (hapten specific) and T (carrier specific) components of the immune response must occur to demonstrate the booster phenomenon.

CELLS INVOLVED IN THE IMMUNE RESPONSE

Characteristic	B Cells	T Cells
Receptor for E.B. Virus	+	−
Binding of Specific Antigen	+	+
Increased in Secondary Response (Memory cells)	+	+
Complement receptor (EAC rosette)	+	−
Site of gamma globulin synthesis	+	−
Phytohemagglutinin (PHA) receptor	−	+
Concanavalin A receptor	−	+
Pokeweed receptor	+	+
LPS receptor	+	−

The secondary response to the injection of an immunogen is called the

_____ response.

The lymphocyte that has a membrane receptor for PHA is the T/B cell.

Receptors for complement components are found in the membranes of

1. B cells.

2. T cells.

3. Macrophages and PMNs.

4. All of the above

5. 1 and 3 only

[answer on next page]

HYBRIDOMAS
  Hybridomas are artificially created cells that produce pure or "monoclonal" antibodies. Having a constant and uniform source of pure antibody, instead of the usual mixture produced by the immune system, not only affords a powerful research tool but can be expected to provide quicker and more accurate diagnosis of viruses, bacteria, and cancer cells. The long-range promise of monoclonal antibodies is that they will be therapeutically useful as vaccine replacement and in the treatment of cancers.

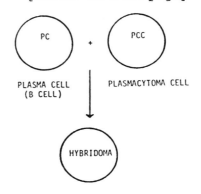

	Cell	SURFACE ANTIGENS ON THYMOCYTE (T CELL) SUBCLASSES				
		Memory	Helper	Cytotoxic	Suppressor	DTH
Antigen	CD4	+	+	−	−	+
	CD8	−	−	+	+	−

CD2 and CD3 are on all peripheral T cells; CD2 functions as an adhesion molecule to hold cells together, CD3 is involved in signal transduction following antigen recognition by T cell receptor/CD4 or CD8 complex.

IMMUNOPROLIFERATIVE DISEASES (MONOCLONAL GAMMOPATHIES) involve an overproduction of immunoglobulins or their fragments by a single clone of plasma cells;

Multiple myeloma - most cases involve IgG. Bence-Jones protein (dimer of light chains) may be found in urine.

Waldenstrom's macroglobulinemia involves IgM overproduction.

Heavy chain disease involves production of incomplete heavy chains. The most common is alpha heavy chain (IgA) disease characterized by intestinal lymphoma.

Amyloidosis in some patients is due to deposition of variable domain fragments of light chains in various organs (e.g kidney).

Cryoglobulinemia and pyroglobulinemia, commonly associated with multiple myeloma, indicate presence of, usually, abnormal IgM molecules in the blood which precipitate at low temperature (cryoglobulins) or high temperature (pyroglobulins).

GENETICS OF THE IMMUNE RESPONSE

Immunoglobulin Specificity
There are three genes involved in synthesis of a light chain, 1 each for the variable, constant and joining regions (V, C, and J respectively). These are selected from a large "library" of genes linked on the same chromosome. There are four genes involved in the synthesis of a heavy chain, V, C, J, and D (for diversity). These also are selected from a large gene pool and re-arranged to serve as an mRNA template.

T Cell Receptor Specificity
Similar genetic selection and rearrangement occurs in T cells during their immunologic maturation. The result of this process is an immunologically specific (epitope specific) receptor in the membrane of the mature T cell.

Immunologic Diversity
The enormous array of reactivities is made possible by the following:
1. multiple genes
2. genomic recombination
3. imprecise joining of V-J, etc.
4. somatic mutations (especially in V gene hypervariable regions)

Review of the Genetics of Immunoglobulin Synthesis

On line 1 the germline chromosomal segment(s) for the mu heavy chain are diagrammed. One each of the many V region genes is selected and linked through rearrangement to selected D and J region genes. This trigenic complex codes for the variable portion of the mu chain. It is transcribed, along with the appropriate C region genes to form the mRNA, which serves as the template for the mu chain polypeptide. After transcription a section or irrelevant RNA [the intron segment] is spliced out to form the functional messenger RNA.

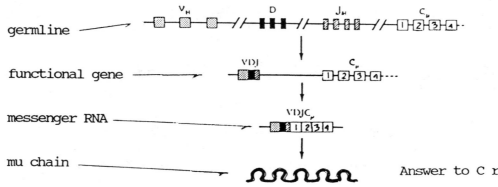

Light chain genes have a similar structure but are on a different chromosome and lack the D region.

Answer to C receptor question = 4

82

IMMUNOSUPPRESSION

IMMUNE SUPPRESSION AND TOLERANCE

Unresponsiveness - the absence of an immune response to a substance that under ordinary conditions would be antigenic. The substance has all the features necessary for antigenicity, but there is no immune response to it. Unresponsiveness can be divided into two broad categories, (1) tolerance, and (2) immunosuppression. The first is antigen specific; in the second, immunosuppression, the host is in a state of general immunologic impairment, i.e., limited or absent response to many antigens.

Natural or autotolerance is the inability to mount an immune response to one's own antigens. Immune tolerance is an artificially induced state of immunologic unresponsiveness to other antigens. Factors which influence the establishment of this state include:

1. Age - the younger the animal, the more easily it is rendered tolerant.
2. Immune status - Obviously correlated with (1) above. However, adults can be rendered tolerant if first immunosuppressed by X-ray or drugs.
3. Amount of Antigen - Less antigen is required to induce T cell tolerance than B cell tolerance.
4. Nature of Antigen - the simpler the antigen, the more efficient it is as a tolerogen. Haptens alone are often good tolerogens; polysaccharides with only a few determinant groups are also effective. Viruses and bacterial cells are very poor tolerogenic materials, as are complex proteins (particularly in aggregated form) due primarily to their antigenic omplexity and ready interaction with phagocytic cells.

The loss of the capacity to make an immune response might be due to deletion of Ag-reactive B cells or T cells or to generation of suppressor cells.

General immunosuppression is encountered in many natural states, including malignancy, senility, developmental difficulty (e.g., diGeorge syndrome) and certain

Cancer patients who are receiving chemotherapy are often susceptible to opportunistic infections. This is due a state of General/Specific immune suppression.

The state of antigen (epitope) specifi immune tolerance is most easily induced in T/B cells?

Autoimmune diseases occur because the body has bypassed the natural state of

_____.

Molecules which interfere with DNA synthesis should be GOOD/BAD general immunosuppressants.

General immunosuppression is encounter in the following natural conditions:

1. _____
2. _____
3. _____
4. _____

infectious diseases such as measles, where a transient loss of cell mediated immunity may be observed. In addition, perinatal removal of the central lymphoid organs (thymus and bursa or its equivalent in mammals - Bone marrow or GALT = gut associated lymphoid tissues) produces deficits in cellular and humoral immunity, respectively. Some immunologists regard mammalian bone marrow as the bursa equivalent.

Immunosuppression may also be induced by chemical or biological treatment regimens, unfortunately often similar to those used in the treatment of autoimmune diseases and cancer.

IMMUNOSUPPRESSIVE AGENTS

A. Lymphotoxic agents - include (1) alkylating agents such as nitrogen mustard and Cytoxan, (2) steroids such as hydrocortisone and prednisone, and (3) X-irradiation. All these agents destroy lymphocytes by damaging their DNA so that their replication is inhibited. (Corticosteroids are thought to have an additional anti-inflammatory action by stabilizing lysosomal membranes.)

B. Anti-metabolites - include such things as purine analogs, pyrimidine analogs and folic acid antagonists. They damage the DNA of lymphoid cells so that they can't divide and become Ab-forming cells. The specificity of all these pharmaceutical agents and X-rays is not directed toward lymphoid cells per se, simply toward rapidly dividing, DNA-synthesizing cells.

C. Antibiotics - Cyclosporin A has recently been shown to be a highly potent immunosuppressive agent. It interferes with IL-2 gene transcription-activating DNA-binding proteins thus inhibiting IL-2 production, preventing T cell growth and development of effector functions.

Answers to questions at top right side of page:

1 = B	2 = A, C	3 = A, C
4 = A, C	5 = A, C	

D. Antibodies - used to inhibit immune
responses in two ways. The first kind of
antibodies are Ab that react with lymphoid
cells. This is the means of attacking
peripheral lymphoid tissue to produce
immunosuppression. Antilymphocyte serum,
particularly antithymocyte serum, is most
useful in transplantation patients; it
is lympholytic.

　　There is another use of Ab in immune
suppression. If preformed Ab is injected
into an animal, followed by injection of
that particular Ag, Ab formation in the
host will be blocked. The injected Ab
binds the injected Ag, and prevents access
of lymphoid tissue to that injected Ag.
This is the principle through which Rhogam
was developed to combat the Rh incompatibility problem. Ab against the
immunogen (Rh° antigen) will neutralize
the Ag through some mechanism, either by
neutralizing the Ag or by coating it in
such a way that its cleared very rapidly.
Thus there is a very short time of access
of Ag to the lymphoid tissue, which would
respond were it not for the injected Ab.
Maternal antibody in a newborn prevents
optimal priming immediately after birth
for the corresponding antigen.

In the table at the bottom of this
sheet, why was there no serious consequence of the Rh- infant born as a
result of the second pregnancy?
(answer on next page)

| PREGNANCY | Rh ANTIGEN PROFILE | | TREATMENT | CONSEQUENCES |
	MOTHER	INFANT		
FIRST	Rh+	Rh-	NONE	NONE
	Rh-	Rh+	NONE	NONE, but mother may become sensitized to Rh antigen during birth process
	Rh-	Rh+	RhoGAM	NONE, and Rh antigen sensitization will NOT occur.
SECOND (et seq.)	Rh-	Rh+	NONE	Infant may develop hemolytic disease (erythroblastosis fetalis), due to maternal IgG destroying Rh+ RBCs of the child.
	Rh-	Rh-	NONE	NONE
	Rh-	Rh+	RhoGAM after 1st birth	NONE

85

SEROLOGIC REACTIONS

ANTIGEN:ANTIBODY REACTIONS

1. The antigen - antibody complex is held together by non-covalent bonding. It will dissociate spontaneously, although the association constant is very high (e.g., 1×10^9 for insulin: anti-insulin interaction).
2. Two main electrostatic forces act to hold the complex together:
   A. Van der Waals forces (act due to spatial fit).
   B. Coulombic forces: electrostatic interactions between positive and negative charges.

If one plots on a graph the antibody-antigen precipitate versus the amount of antigen added to a fixed amount of antibody, one notices the following:

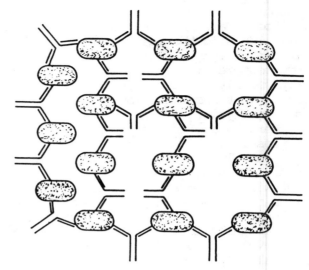

Lattice structure of antigen-antibody reactions.

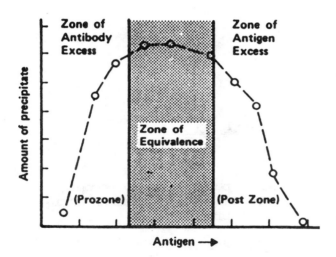

Agglutination occurs if the antigen is particulate (e.g., _____ or _____; see next page). Precipitation is the result of antibody reacting with soluble antigens such as serum albumin.

Where the antigen concentration is very low with a relative superabundance of antibody (Zone of Ab excess), formation of complexes occurs but residual Ab will remain in the supernatant. This area is known as a prozone. As more antigen is added, the antibody (AB) - antigen (Ag) complex forms a precipitate due to the production of a lattice of molecules which forms a large network (Zone of Equivalence) but instead of reaching a plateau this curve comes back down to zero with increasing amounts of antigen (Zone of Ag excess).

<u>Answer to question from preceding page</u>
The infant's RBCs do not contain the Rh Ag in their membranes therefore they will not be sensitized to complement-mediated lysis or erythrophagocytosis by the anti-Rh IgG antibodies that have passively crossed the placenta.

When a zone of Ab excess occurs in vivo the precipitates are usually removed from the circulation very rapidly (A process known as immune elimination). The antigen usually remains in the body long enough to effect a booster to the pre-existing immune system. However, in instances of passively acquired antibody, no priming or immunologic memory may result (e.g., Rhogam intervention of Rh sensitization, pooled gamma globulin prophylaxis for rubella and hepatitis).

When Ag excess occurs in vivo it may result in a disease called serum sickness. An example of this would be the administration of snake venom antitoxin contained in horse serum, which to a human is a foreign protein. Some persons develop serum sickness. The soluble Ag-Ab complex causes the release of various mediators with resultant vasculitis, urticaria, etc. Immune complexes probably account for most glomerulonephritis in man.

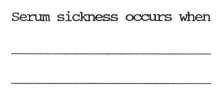

Serum sickness occurs when

_____

_____

_____.

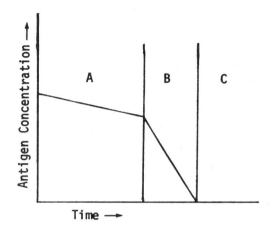

A = Normal catabolism phase of antigen clearance.
B = Immune clearance phase; Ag:Ab complexes form here.
C = phase of detectable antibody.

REACTIONS OF VARIOUS CLASSES OF IMMUNOGLOBULINS

Reaction	IgG	IgA	IgM
Agglutination	+	+	++
Precipitation	+	+	+
Virus neutralization	+	+	+
C fixation	++	−	+
C dependent lysis	+	−	+++
Immune Complex	++	−	+

The immunoglobulin class which is the

most efficient at "fixing" complement is

IgG/IgM. The IgG/IgM excels at

sensitizing cells for C dependent lysis.

[answer to question from preceding page: bacterial cells or erythrocytes, i.e., hemagglutination]

RADIOIMMUNOASSAY

Radioimmunoassay (RIA) is an extremely sensitive method that can be used for the quantitation of any substance that (1) is antigenic or haptenic and (2) can be labeled with a radioactive isotope, for example, I^{125}. The method is capable of measuring picogram quantities or less, depending on the substance being assayed. Basically, the method depends upon the competition between labeled (known) and unlabeled (unknown) antigen for the same antibody. A known amount of labeled antigen, a known amount of specific antibody, and an unknown amount of unlabeled antigen are allowed to react together. The antigen-antibody complexes that form are then separated out, and their radioactivity is determined. By measuring the radioactivity still remaining in the supernatant (unbound, labeled antigen), one can calculate the percentage of labeled antigen bound to the antibody. The concentration of an unknown (unlabeled) antigen can be determined by reference to a standard curve constructed from data obtained by allowing varying amounts of unlabeled antigen to compete.

Energy (E) emitted from labeled Ab is detected by scintillation counter.

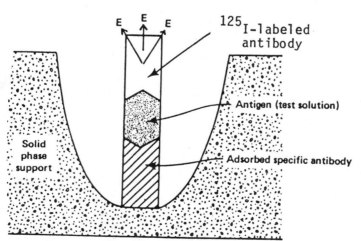

Relative sensitivity of serological procedures to detect antibody

most sensitive = RIA

ELISA

AGGLUTINATION

FLOCCULATION

least sensitive = PRECIPITATION

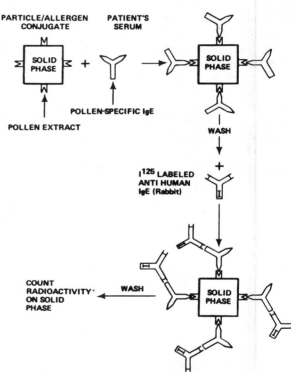

The above diagram depicts a RAST (radioallergosorbent test) used to quantitate the amount of allergen specific IgE in the serum of an atopic person. The PRIST (paper radioimmunosorbent test) measures total IgE. It employs anti-IgE as the "capture" ligand in the solid phase.

ENZYME-LINKED IMMUNOSORBENT ASSAY

Enzyme-linked Immunosorbent Assay (ELISA) has virtually the same sensitivity as radioimmunoassay. It can be used to assay both antigens and antibodies. The requisites are (1) the antigen or antibody can be attached to a solid phase support and still retain its immunological activity (2) either antigen or antibody can be linked to an enzyme and (3) both immunological and enzymatic activity are retained by the antigen- or antibody-enzyme complex. Solid phase support systems used include paper disks, plastic surfaces, etc.; enzymes used include horseradish peroxidase and alkaline phosphatase. The application of one variant of ELISA, the double antibody sandwich for the assay of an antigen, is performed as follows. Antibody specific for the antigen being assayed is coated on a plastic surface (polystyrene plate). The solution being tested for antigen is applied to the surface, and any unreacted material is removed by washing. Enzyme-labeled specific antibody is then applied , and any excess conjugate is removed by washing. Finally, the enzyme substrate is added. The rate of substrate degradation is determined by the amount of enzyme-labeled antibody bound, which is determined by the amount of antigen in the solution being tested. A substrate that will give a color change on degradation is chosen. The color change can be measured quantitatively in a spectrophotometer.

These assays are VERY sensitive and have been used to detect microbial antigens in body fluids. For example, detection of Haemophilus influenzae type b or cryptococcal capsular polysaccharides in spinal fluid, or streptococcal group A specific carbohydrate antigen in cell extracts.

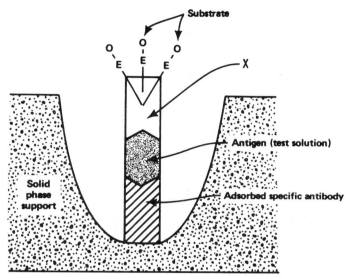

In the figure above what is the substance labeled "X"?

(answer at bottom of page)

X = Enzyme-labeled specific antibody

89

THE COOMBS TEST

Various factors are involved in the detection of antibodies against the Rh antigens. These antibodies, commonly seen in erythroblastosis fetalis, are able to cause agglutination in the presence of high concentrations of proteins, or if the erythrocyte has previously been stripped of certain cell membrane constituents by mild enzyme treatment. If such conditions are not fulfilled, the antibodies will not agglutinate the red blood cells, but will still attach to them. This adsorbed gamma globulin can be detected by the addition of an antiserum against human gamma globulin prepared in a non-human mammal (Coombs serum). The Coombs test can be used to detect hemolytic disease of the newborn, hemolytic transfusion reactions, idiopathic acquired hemolytic anemia, and autoimmune hemolytic anemia.

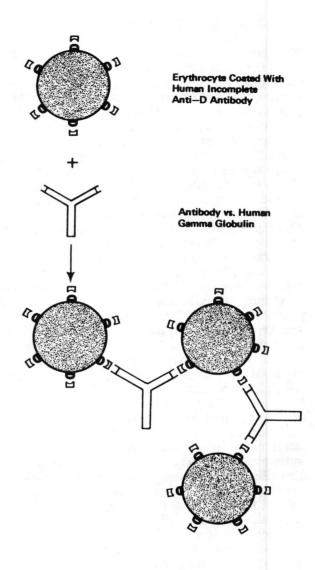

Erythrocyte Coated With
Human Incomplete
Anti—D Antibody

Antibody vs. Human
Gamma Globulin

In the assay to the right, if the antibody were tagged with fluorescein it could also be used in:

1. SLE to detect Ab vs DNA.

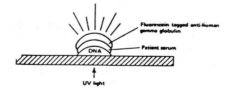

Fluorescein tagged anti-human gamma globulin

Patient serum

DNA

UV light

2. syphilis to detect Ab vs T. pallidum (FTA test)

HYPERSENSITIVITY REACTIONS

IMMEDIATE HYPERSENSITIVITY

The manifestations of immediate hypersensitivity are not protective, but rather are deleterious. There is genetic predisposition toward atopic (Type I, Gell and Coombs) hypersensitivity. The Type I hypersensitivities manifest themselves in many different ways, depending on the target organ. Some of these manifestations are:

1. <u>Anaphylaxis</u> - an immediate hypersensitivity reaction which causes bronchoconstriction in humans. The main symptom is the inability to breathe; there is complete vasomotor collapse and bronchoconstriction.

2. <u>Allergic asthma</u> (extrinsic asthma) - characterized mainly by bronchospasm. Eosinophilia in blood and sputum may be seen.

3. <u>Allergic rhinitis</u> (hay fever) - characterized mainly by watery nasal discharge, sneezing, etc. Eosinophilia may be present in nasal secretions.

4. <u>Allergic urticaria</u> (hives) - characterized by wheals (dermal edema), erythema (reddening), angioedema (severe local swelling) around the face and sometimes respiratory obstruction due to edema in the larynx and pharynx.

5. <u>Atopic dermatitis</u> (eczema) - characterized by pruritis (itching), usually seen in infants or young children.

Some of the manifestations of ATOPIC

disease are:

1. _____

2. _____

3. _____

4. _____

5. _____

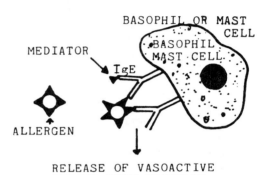

RELEASE OF VASOACTIVE
AMINES FROM GRANULES

* ANAPHYLAXIS
* BRONCHOSPASM
* EDEMA

COMPLETE THE TABLE BELOW (It will be necessary to read ahead)

Gell and Coombs Classification	Immune Reactivity	Mechanism of Tissue Damage
TYPE I		
TYPE II		
TYPE III		
TYPE IV		

The primary class of antibodies that cause allergic responses in man is IgE. IgE is a noncomplement fixing, non-placental passing antibody that has a re markable tissue affinity (homocytotropic). It binds in tissue to the mast cell and to the basophil in blood, via the Fc fragment. The small amount of IgE in the serum is of major importance in that it is responsible for a passive cutaneous test for the detection of allergies (Prausnitz-Kustner or P-K test) and the very sensitive RIA tests (RAST & PRIST).

When an allergen attaches to the combining sites of the antibody, the mast cell or basophil is triggered to degranulate and release a number of different biologically active materials. This process is energy-requiring, requires the bridging of two cell-bound IgE molecules by allergen, and does not involve cell death. The materials are biologically active mediators and are the cause of the symptoms of immediate hypersensitivity. Some of these substances are; 1) histamine, 2) slow reacting substance of anaphylaxis (SRS-A), 3) bradykinin, 4) serotonin, 5) eosinophil chemotactic factor of anaphylaxis, 6) platelet-activating factor, and 7) prostaglandin and leukotriene products of arachadonic acid metabolism. They contract smooth muscle, and increase capillary permeability. Complement is not involved in atopic allergies.

The second type of allergic disease classified by Gell and Coombs (type II) is due to cytotoxic antibodies. The antigen on the cell surface combines with antibody and sensitizes the cell to lysis or phagocytosis. In the presence of complement the C cascade ensues, with destruction of the membrane and generation of chemotactic factors, etc. An example of this type of injury is erythroblastosis fetalis (see page 99). Other examples of type II hypersensitivity are autoimmune hemolytic disease and Goodpasture's Syndrome.

Allergen reactions with mast cell-bound IgE causes the following sequence of events:
1) Influx of Ca^{++}
2) Protease activation
3) Decrease in cAMP
4) Granule margination and fusion with the membrane
5) Exocytosis of granule contents

Cromolyn sodium stabilizes lysosomal membranes of mast cells and prevents degranulation and release of histamine and other pharmacologically active mediators of atopic disease.

Pharmacologic mediators of atopy include:

1. _____
2. _____
3. _____
4. _____
5. _____
6. _____
7. _____
8. _____

Complement is/is not involved in atopic allergies.

IMMUNE-COMPLEX DISEASE
(TYPE III REACTION OF GELL AND COOMBS)

In experimental animals there is an induced disease called the Arthus reaction. It is similar to serum sickness; they both have the same trigger, i.e., administration of foreign serum or drugs. The symptoms are fever, lymph node enlargement, a rash, and arthritis. The mechanism is as follows: Antibody of the IgM or IgG type is produced against the foreign protein. When the level of Ab is significant enough to form Ag-Ab complexes, there is still an Ag excess. The complexes at this point are soluble and cause the ensuing · process to occur. The Ag-Ab complex activates the complement system and this Ag-Ab-C complex is deposited primarily in the basement membrane of the glomerulus of the kidney. PMN leukocytes are chemotactically attracted to the site of deposition of the complex by the C5a chemotaxin. They proceed to release their lysosomal enzymes into the extracellular space, and their proteolytic enzymes destroy the basement membrane with the resulting symptoms of kidney failure. A similar process occurs in the other tissues (synovial membranes, vascular endothelium). Serum complement levels may be decreased. A hallmark of the disease is the "lumpy-bumpy" deposit of complexes on the membrane revealed by immunofluorescence.

Serum sickness is not the only example of immune complex injury. Any time there is an antigen that triggers production of antigen-antibody-complement complexes that ends up in the joints or the kidney, there will be a case of immune complex disease. Two examples are:
1) post-streptococcal glomerulonephritis and
2) nephritis of systemic lupus erythematosus.

Examples of cytotoxic antibody-mediated diseases include:

1. _____

2. _____

3. _____

> Toxic immune complexes form in the region of antigen excess, i.e., at the beginning of an immune response.

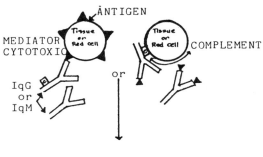

What type of immunologic injury is depicted in the illustration above?

Immune complex deposition in the glomeruli would be evidenced by a (lumpy-bumpy/linear) pattern of immunofluorescence along the basement membrane if the kidney is stained with a fluorescein-tagged antibody specific for human (gamma globulin/complement/either).

93

DELAYED HYPERSENSITIVITY

Cellular immunity (delayed hypersensitivity) is a reaction involving the T lymphocyte. It has nothing to do with circulating antibodies. The histologic hallmark of delayed hypersensitivity is an accumulation of mononuclear cells (lymphocytes and monocytes) at the site of the reaction causing induration.

Delayed hypersensitivity is especially characteristic of many chronic microbial infections, and in particular those that are intracellular. Tuberculosis, brucellosis and typhoid fever are examples where the immunity is based on cellular events. Protection from fungal infections (histoplasmosis, blastomycosis), and virtually all viral infections is due to cellular immunity. Specifically-sensitized lymphocytes can destroy virus-infected cells, as can antibody plus complement. Some disease manifestations of fungi are due to delayed hypersensitivity and, while circulating antibodies are also demonstrable in viral infections, recovery from viral infections is primarily cellular whereas resistance to re-infection is usually antibody-mediated. Graft rejection, tumor immunity and some autoimmune diseases also have a strong cell-mediated immunity component.

The T cell antigen receptor (that part of the membrane which imparts immunologic specificity to the cell) is structurally very similar to an Fab molecule, although chemically quite different. The antigen receptor has 2 polypeptide chains, alpha and beta, both of which contain constant and variable domains. The chains also contain short J and D regions, further mirroring the structure of the antigen binding portion of antibody molecules.

Examples of immune complex induced disease include:

1. _____

2. _____

3. _____

Cell-mediated immunity is a common feature of infections by

1. _____

2. _____

3. _____

4. _____

5. _____

Answer: The illustration is of Gell and Coombs Type II immune injury by the action of cytotoxic antibodies.

In Goodpasture's disease, antibody deposition in the glomeruli would be evidenced by (lumpy-bumpy/linear) pattern of immunofluorescence along the basement membrane if the kidney is stained with a fluorescein tagged antibody specific for human gamma globulin/complement/either.

The activated T cell involved in cell-mediated immunity has the following characteristics.

1. It is cytotoxic. Following a homograft, the host makes sensitized lymphocytes which destroy the graft in the absence of immunosuppressant therapy. The suppression of the sensitized T cell is a <u>must</u> for successful transplantation.

2. It produces a substance known as Transfer Factor, or TF, which, like T cells, can transfer passively this type of reactivity to another host or to neighboring cells. TF can cause the activation of new T cells.

3. It produces many soluble factors called lyphokines, migration inhibitory factor (MIF), macrophage activating factor (MAF), macrophage chemotactic factor, mitogenic factor for lymphocytes, lymphotoxin, leukocyte inhibitory factor, etc.

Other forms of Type IV reactivity include contact (e.g., poison ivy, DNCB sensitivity) and certain drug allergies. Here, the inducing agents act as haptens and become antigenic via coupling to host proteins.

<u>Products of Activated Lymphocytes</u>

Mediators affecting macrophages
 Migration inhibitory factor (MIF)
 Macrophage activating factor (MAF)
 Chemotactic factor for macrophages
 (MCF)
Mediators affecting polymorphonuclear
 leukocytes
 Leukocyte inhibitory factor (LIF)
 Chemotactic factors for neutrophils,
 eosinophils, and basophils
Mediators affecting lymphocytes
 Mitogenic factors
 Immunoregulatory factors
 Transfer factor (TF)
Factors affecting other cell types
 Lymphotoxins
 Growth inhibitory factors
 Osteoclast-activating factor
 Interferon
 Colony stimulating activity
 Perforins

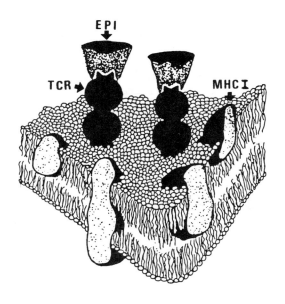

The reaction illustrated above will result in the release of what lymphokines? [list only the 6 most important]

1) _____

2) _____

3) _____

4) _____

5) _____

6) _____

MANY OF THE ACTIVITIES LISTED TO THE LEFT ARE DUE TO FACTORS CALLED <u>INTERLEUKINS</u>. AT THE PRESENT THERE ARE AT LEAST TEN IL-1, IL-2, etc. MOST ARE THE PRODUCT OF T CELLS [cf "Review Statements" for more details].

AUTOIMMUNITY

AUTOIMMUNE DISEASES

Autoimmune diseases are defined as the occurrence of an immune response resulting in the production of either antibody and/or sensitized lymphoid cells capable of reacting with normal body constituents. There are several hypothesized mechanisms for the development of autoimmune disease.

1. Release of a sequestered antigen which then induce an immune response.

2. Self antigens may be slightly altered and thus become immunogenic.

3. Cross-reacting (heterophile) or closely related antigen. For example, streptococci and human heart tissue share a common antigen.

4. The spontaneous emergence of clones of cells ("forbidden clones") capable of making an immune response to one's own tissues.

5. Deficiency of suppressor T cells (an immunodeficiency disease that results in autoimmunity).

There are several general signs of autoimmune disease. These include:

1. Increase in the amount of serum gamma globulin.

2. Occurence of different autoantibodies.

3. Decreased concentration of complement in serum.

4. Presence of immune complexes in serum.

5. Absence of T8 lymphocytes (this is a membrane marker of T suppressor cells).

6. Lumpy-bumpy immunoglobulin and C deposits seen in immune complex diseases in vascular walls and basement membranes.

7. Linear deposit of immunoglobulin and complement in anti-glomerular basement membrane diseases such as Goodpasture's.

General features of autoimmune diseases include:

1. _____

2. _____

3. _____

4. _____

5. _____

6. _____

7. _____

Serum complement levels are depressed during acute episodes of many auto-immune diseases because

A. the macrophages stop synthesizing these proteins
B. the liver produces an excess of C inhibitors such as protein I
C. these proteins are consumed in the immune complexes
D. these proteins are preferentially catabolized and excreted by the kidney

(answer on next page)

POST-VACCINAL ENCEPHALOMYELITIS

Post-vaccinal encephalomyelitis (PVE), first seen in an occasional individual given rabies vaccine, follows the injection of nervous tissue. It may occur following immunization with embryo-derived vaccines. In man, the signs and symptoms usually appear in one week to 10 days following subcutaneous injection and include:

1. Irritation at the site of injection with induration, inflammation and sometimes pain, progressing to headache and backache.
2. Paralysis and general weakness in the extremities. There is demyelination and accumulations of cells around blood vessels, a perivascular "cuffing." These cells are lymphocytes, and this is a cellular type response.

This disease, with all its signs and symptoms, has been reproduced in animals where it is called experimental allergic encephalomelitis. A highly purified basic protein (made up of basic amino acids), a histone-like protein, has been identified as the responsible antigen in nervous tissue.

There are several other human diseases similar to post-vaccinal encephalomyelitis. One of them occurs following measles (subacute sclerosing panencephalitis or SSPE) and is a virus-induced disease whose mechanism is unknown. Another is multiple sclerosis.

THYROIDITIS

This disease involves the antigen, thyroglobulin. Several kinds of antibodies are made in response to this antigen. In the target organ, the thyroid, there is an accumulation of lymphoid cells which somehow have the ability to disrupt the colloid of the gland causing fibrosis.

Although thyroglobulin is the major antigen identified with this disease, two other antigens have been found within thyroid tissue. Thyroiditis has been passively transferred to normal hosts by sensitized lymphocytes and serum.

The absence of T suppressor cells in certain patients with autoimmune disease is detected by enumerating the number of cells bearing the CD4/CD8 membrane marker.

Three central nervous system diseases

which resemble post-vaccinal encephalitis

are:

1. _____

2. _____

3. _____

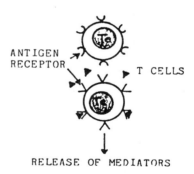

ANTIGEN RECEPTOR

T CELLS

RELEASE OF MEDIATORS

(answer to question on preceding page = C)

SYSTEMIC LUPUS ERYTHEMATOSUS

Systemic lupus erythematosus (SLE), is a generalized autoimmune disease; virtually all organs in the body appear to be affected, though most fatalities in this disease appear to have the kidney as the target organ. This disease predominates in women, 10-40 years of age.

The hallmark of SLE is the LE cell, or lupus erythematosus cell, which is a polymorphonuclear leukocyte which has phagocytized some nuclear material. It may appear as an inclusion body with the cell's own nucleus pushed to the side.

The conclusion from this observation is that SLE involves an immune response against nuclear protein or nuclear material, causing its extrusion from the cell. However, antibodies are directed against several targets:

1. nucleoprotein
2. nucleoli
3. DNA
4. Ro, La, Sm antigens
5. RBC and platelets
6. gamma globulins
7. mitochondria
8. clotting factors

The renal failure that leads to death seems to be due to immune complex disease. The renal damage is attributable to immune complexes consisting of DNA plus the antibody, and complement; these complexes are deposited in the glomeruli causing destruction or dissolution of the basement membrane. Serum complement levels are often depressed.

Several patterns of nuclear staining are seen in this disease. Homogenous staining is due to anti-DNA antibodies; the outline pattern will be produced by anti-dsDNA antibodies or antibodies against soluble nucleoprotein. Both these patterns are characteristic of ACTIVE SLE disease. The speckled pattern reflects the presence of antibodies to non-DNA nuclear components. High levels of these antibodies is indicative of mixed connective tissue disease. The nucleolar pattern of staining is most often seen in sceroderma and polymyositis. Numerous other autoimmune diseases may present with anti-nuclear staining reactions (e.g., Rheumatoid arthritis, Sjogren's).

SLE is one of the classic autoimmune diseases, affecting approximately 1 per 1,000 in the U.S. Many diverse autoantibodies are seen in these patients, including antibodies against

1. _____

2. _____

3. _____

4. _____

5. _____

6. _____

7. _____

8. _____

The importance of complement in SLE glomerulonephritis is as a chemotactic stimulus. A significant infiltration of PMNs is seen and these cells are responsible for most of the tissue damage due to the release of hydrolytic enzyme and other mediator molecules which cause local damage.

AUTOIMMUNE HEMOLYTIC DISEASE

Autoimmune hemolytic disease (AHD) involves the destruction of one's own RBC's. Some of the antibodies involved are incomplete or non-agglutinating and can be detected only with Coomb's serum (Ab against human gamma globulin). Two types of antibodies are found in AHD: warm antibodies and cold antibodies. These antibodies are not exclusively found with AHD; for example, cold antibodies have been identified with mycoplasmal pneumonia. The mechanism of this disease is unknown but involves destruction of RBC's.

The following is a list of diseases which are also thought to have an auto-immune etiology:

1. Idiopathic Addison's disease in which antibody is formed to the adrenal gland.
2. Rheumatoid arthritis involves rheumatoid factor (RF) which is mainly IgM antibody. This antibody is formed against another immunoglobulin, IgG. These people are making an immune response to their own IgG.
3. Guillain-Barre (acute idiopathic polyneuritis) in which sensitized lymphocytes are formed against peripheral nervous tissue - peripheral neuritis.
4. Idiopathic thrombocytopenic purpura in which antibodies are made against blood platelets.
5. Myasthenia gravis - antibody and sensitized lymphocytes against acetyl choline receptors.
6. Goodpasture's syndrome - antibody which cross reacts with alveolar and glomerular basement membranes.
7. Pernicious anemia - antibody against parietal cells and/or intrinsic factor.
8. Insulin dependent diabetes mellitus - antibody and sensitized T cells against insulin-producing beta cells in the islets of Langerhans.

Match the autoimmune disease with the antigen.

1. Addison's disease

2. Guillain Barre

3. Rheumatoid arthritis

4. Myasthenia gravis

5. Goodpasture's syndrome

6. Systemic lupus erythematosus

7. Pernicious anemia

   A. DNA

   B. Adrenal gland

   C. Basement membrane

   D. Peripheral nervous tissue

   E. IgG

   F. Intrinsic factor

   G. Acetyl choline receptors

(answers below, left)

1 = B	5 = C
2 = D	6 = A
3 = E	7 = F
4 = G	

IMMUNE DEFICIENCY DISEASES

TESTS TO DETERMINE IMMUNE FUNCTION

Phagocytic cells = Phagocytosis, intra-cellular killing, chemotaxis, nitroblue tetrazolium reduction

B cells = Ig levels, isohemagglutinins, typhoid agglutinins, Schick test, allergy scratch test, EAC rosettes

T cells = PHA stimulation, SRBC rosettes, DNCB sensitization, skin test with common antigens, e.g. Candida, trichophytin, streptokinase- streptodornase (varidase)

DEFICIENCIES IN NON-SPECIFIC RESISTANCE

Two inherited diseases which cause decreased production of effective phago-cytic cells at the bone marrow level are: (1) Reticular dysgenesis affects all stem cells by drastically diminishing their production.
(2) The Fanconi syndrome (or congenital pancytopenia) has as its signs the suppression of erythroid blood elements (the patient has an anemia), and suppres-sion of the myeloid series (polymorpho-nuclear leukocytes or PMN's).

Also important are diseases which affect the functions of phagocytic cells instead of affecting the numbers of these cells.

Chronic Granulomatous Disease is char-acterized by recurrent, primarily bacterial, infections. The mechanism is a defect in the oxidized NAD - related activities, (deficiency of NADH or NADPH oxidase) in the PMN's.

Neutrophils from patients with Chediak-Higashi syndrome have deficiencies in chemotaxis and intracellular killing.

Complement deficiencies may also predispose an individual to recurrent bacterial infections. The most severe are deficiencies of C3 and C5, which are the complement components most closely associated with native immune mechanisms (opsonization and chemotaxis). Absence of late components [C5-9] is associated with severe meningococcal infections.

THE MOST IMPORTANT HALLMARK OF IMMUNODEFICIENCY IS THE OCCURRENCE OF REPEATED INFECTIONS, OFTEN BY ORGANISMS CONSIDERED TO BE OF LOW VIRULENCE.

The major immunologic features of chronic granulomatous disease are:

1. Occurrence of recurrent infections with organisms of low virulence, e.g., S. epidermidis, Aspergillus, Serratia.

2. X-linked inheritance (a female variant does occur rarely).

3. Onset of infections occurs by 2 years of age.

4. Diseases = pneumonia, osteomyelitis, abscesses

5. Diagnosis established by nitroblue tetrazolium test or intracellular killing assay of peripheral blood neutrophils.

100

DEFICIENCIES IN SPECIFIC RESISTANCE

Thymic-independent areas. This refers to the bursa equivalent, or a defect in the B cell, the plasma cell, or the production of the five classes of immunoglobulins, e.g., Bruton's congenital hypogammaglobulinemia. The patient has recurrent bacterial infections especially pneumonias, otitis media, etc. There may be no detectable immunoglobulins in the serum. Their cellular immune system is intact and therefore, the patient can reject tissue grafts, become tuberculin positive and resist fungal and viral infection (with the possible exception of polio). They have no germinal centers in their lymph nodes, and no plasma cells in the lymph nodes, spleen, or marrow. Tonsillar and Peyer's Patch tissues are either hypoplastic or absent. There are normal levels of circulating lymphocytes due to the fact that most of these are T cells. The treatment is administration of pooled gamma globulin.

Selective Immunoglobulin Deficiency is a syndrome in which there are isolated deficiencies of any one or two classes of immunoglobulins. The most common is IgA. These patients may have repeated infections of the sinopulmonary or gastrointestinal systems.

Thymic dependent areas. The Di George syndrome (thymic hypoplasia) is the absence of the thymus due to the faulty development of the third and fourth pharyngeal pouches in the embryo. The patient has no cellular immunity, but has normal levels of plasma cells and circulating antibodies.

Nezelof Syndrome is a deficiency in thymus accompanied by selective immunoglobulin deficiency. These patients are unable to respond to immunogenic stimuli.

Chronic mucocutaneous candidiasis is a T cell abnormality with no skin test response to Candida. The patients usually expire of endocrinopathy.

Bruton's disease is an X-linked condition, which means it is seen in males/females.

The major immunologic features of Bruton's X-linked hypogammaglobulinemia are:

1. recurrent pyogenic infections beginning at 5-6 mo.
2. Absence of B cells in peripheral blood.
3. Absence of germinal centers.
4. IgG less than 200 mg/dl.
5. Absence of other immunoglobulins.
6. Good clinical response to pooled gamma globulins.

The most common immunoglobulin deficiency seen in the "selective" category is a deficiency in _____.

T lymphocyte numbers can be estimated by the following tests:

1. Sheep RBC rosettes
2. Membrane marker stains such as fluorescein-labelled anti-CD2 or CD3.
3. Peripheral blood lymphocyte count (as most are T cells).

T lymphocyte function can be estimated by the following tests:

1. _____
2. _____
3. _____

More serious is the severe combined immunodeficiency (SCID) which involves thymic independent and thymic dependent mechanisms. This is also known as Swiss type agammaglobulinemia. The defect, extremely severe, is in both cellular and humoral immune mechanisms. There is a depression of lymphocytes, plasma cells, circulating antibodies, and delayed hypersensitivity; there are no germinal centers in the lymph nodes; there is little thymus. This disease is usually fatal within the first year or two of life. A biochemical defect (deficiency of the enzyme adenosine deaminase, ADA) has been identified in about 50% of SCID patients with the autosomal recessive form of the disease.

Another purine catabolism enzyme, purine nucleoside phosphorylase, is defective in some infants with T cell deficiencies.

Other disease syndromes are accompanied by deficits in the immune response. One of these is the Wiskott-Aldrich syndrome in which the patients have recurrent infections. They have a general depression in the number of lymphocytes and thrombocytes, and a defect in their cellular immunity and delayed hypersensitivity (because of the low number of lymphocytes). They also have a defect in their ability to produce antibodies to polysaccharide antigens. They do not make normal levels of antibodies, especially IgM.

There is a disease syndrome called ataxia telangiectasia characterized by immune deficiency. These patients have recurrent infections (usually pulmonary), ataxia, general depression of cellular and humoral immunity, with decreased IgA and IgE.

Sarcoidosis, Hodgkin's disease and lepromatous leprosy involve suppression of lymphocytes, which are mandatory for cellular immunity. Other tumors may also cause defects in cellular immunity, as evidenced by lack of reactivity to a battery of commonly encountered Ag's such as PPD, mumps, Candida, streptokinase and streptodornase.

Acquired and secondary immunodeficiency

I. Acquired Immune Deficiency Syndrome (AIDS)

Major features include:

a. Depressed CD4 (helper) lymphocytes which cause inversion of CD4-CD8 ratio; CD4 is the membrane receptor for HIV
b. Reduced lymphocyte response to PHA
c. Increased circulating immune complexes.
d. Reduced NK cell activity.
e. Anti-HIV antibodies in serum.
f. Infections with bizarre opportunists such as Pneumocystis carinii, and other organisms (e.g., cryptococcus, cytomegalovirus, candida, mycobacteria and strongyloides).

II. Secondary Immune Deficiency

a. Due to infections, usually transient and non-specific
   1. Measles
   2. Rubella
   3. Other viral disease
   4. Leprosy*
   5. Tuberculosis*
   6. Coccidioidomycosis*
   *These are usually specific to the agent and last for the duration of the illness.

b. Due to malignancies
   1. Hodgkin's
   2. Leukemia

c. Autoimmune diseases-may be due to therapy

   1. SLE
   2. Rheumatoid arthritis

d. Other conditions
   1. Diabetes
   2. Alcoholism
   3. Sarcoidosis

TRANSPLANTATION IMMUNOLOGY

TERMINOLOGY USED IN TRANSPLANTATION

Autograft - graft from one part of the body to another (e.g. skin)

Allograft (homograft) - graft from one member of a species to another

Xenograft - graft from one species to another Terms used to describe antigenic relationship between donor and recipient

Autologous - same individual: in inbred animals the term is syngeneic

Heterologous - different individuals: allogeneic antigen source or xenogeneic antigen source

In the human, the major histocompatability locus is called the HLA locus (human leucocyte antigen). The alleles are expressed codominately.

Nature of histocompatibility antigens

1. Products of genes of the MHC (major histocompatibility complex)
2. Glycoprotein component of cell membrane
3. Occurs in lymphocytes in high concenttrations; also present on other nucleated cells of the body (e.g., macrophage, hepatocytes)
4. Are divided into 2 classes (see figure at the right)
   a. Class I = coded for by HLA A, B, and C genes; function as target antigens for immune recognition and killing
   b. Class II = coded for by HLA - DR, DQ and DP genes: function as recognition molecules in cellular regulation of immune interaction; found on B cells, macrophages, and activated T cells
   c. Class III = complement components C2, C4 and B are coded for in the MHC region; genes for tumor necrosis factor are also found in the MHC region

A kidney graft between identical twins would be allogeneic/syngeneic.

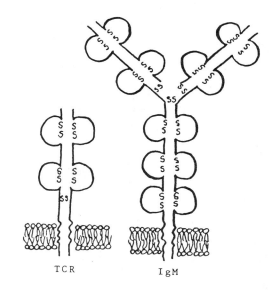

TCR IgM

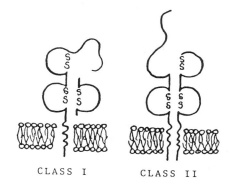

CLASS I CLASS II

NOTE THE STRUCTURAL SIMILARITY TO THE T CELL RECEPTOR AND THE IMMUNOGLOBULIN M MOLECULE THAT ARE DEPICTED IN THE TOP PANEL.

103

Major Histocompatibility Complex restriction

MHC restricton is the requirement that an antigen presenting cell must co-express in its membrane a foreign epitope and a self MHC molecule. Only then can the T cell effectively interact with that cell. The T cell receptor recognizes the epitope and a CD molecule recognizes the MHC protein; CD4 molecules recognize Class II MHC proteins and CD8 molecules recognize Class I MHC proteins.

HOST RESPONSE TO TRANSPLANT

First of all, one can make antibodies to the histocompatibility antigens. One can also get a T-cell activation or cellular immune response. Both of these responses can be mounted following a transplant.

There are at least three types of rejection reactions that can take place following a transplant.

1. Hyperacute rejection - performed ANTI-BODIES attack the organ. There is a rapid vascular spasm and vascular occlusion and the organ is not perfused by recipient's blood.

Hyperacute rejection occurs within hours or days.

2. Acute or Accelerated rejection - this is believed to be due to sensitized T LYMPHOCYTES. This is a type of rejection reaction that one sees 10-30 days after a transplant. Since the patient has not been previously sensitized it takes a while to develop sensitized immune lymphocytes which then increase in number and attack the graft. Here we see the typical picture of a cell-mediated immune response. We see infiltration into the graft (especially around small blood vessels) of small lymphocytes and mononuclear cells along with some granulocytes which causes destruction of the graft transplant.

3. Chronic rejection - in a kidney transplant with this kind of rejection one sees a slow loss of kidney function over a period of months or years. It may be a cellular immune response, an antibody response, or a combination of the two.

The induction of an antibody response requires 1) T cell recognition of the epitope [via the T cell receptor], 2) B cell recognition of the epitope [via membrane-bound IgM], and 3) T cell recognition of the MHC class II protein [via its CD4 molecule.

The expression of T cell cytotoxicity requires 1) T cell recognition of the epitope [via the T cell receptor], 2) T cell recognition of the Class I MHC protein [via its CD8 molecule].

Class I histocompatibility antigens are

coded for by the HLA genes _____

_____. They function as

_____

_____.

Class II histocompatibility antigens are

coded for by the HLA genes _____

_____. They function as

_____

_____.

Class III histocompatibility genes code

for _____.

POSTGRAFT PATIENT MANAGEMENT

All transplants, except between identical twins, require immunosuppression. Drugs, or chemical or physical manipulations are used to reduce the immune and inflammatory responses.

One class of drugs used is the corticosteroids. Other drugs that are used anti-metabolites or alkylating agents such as azthioprine and cyclophosphimide. Cyclosporin A is a fungal product that inhibits helper T cells. Anti-lymphocyte globulin or antithymocyte globulin is also used in the management of the recipient.

With the use of such high doses of immunosuppressive drugs, one often gets into trouble with infection and/or malignancy. About 25% of the deaths that occur in kidney transplants are due to sepsis.

GRAFT VS HOST DISEASE

This is not a problem with heart or kidney transplants but is a problem in bone marrow transplants. The problem occurs in immunologically nonresponsive recipients whenever there is an antigen difference between donor and recipient, such as is the case when parental cells (e.g., AA) are injected into the F_1 (AB) offspring. If the bone marrow (since it produces immunologically competent cells such as lymphocytes) can produce lymphocytes which can become sensitized to the recipient's antigens. Thus, the graft tissue can mount an immunological attack on the recipient. This is graft rejection of the host. The graft vs host reaction in humans is characterized by liver abnormalities, by a skin rash that looks like measles, and by diarrhea, wasting, and death.

Complete the following table.

Type of Rejection	Time of Onset	Immunologic Basis
Hyperacute		
Acute		
Chronic		

Grafts where the donor is a cadaver are

A. aberrant
B. abhorrent
C. allografts
D. dumb
E. illegal

Graft vs. host disease occurs when

_____

_____

_____ .

Symptoms of this phenomenon in humans

include

1. _____

2. _____

3. _____

Bone marrow transplantation has proven to be of value in the therapy of several diseases. The marrow serves as a source of **stem cells**; in some instances replacing a stem cell that nature omitted, in other cases supplying a source of normal precursor cells following chemotherapy for malignancy. Diseases in which bone marrow transplantation has been useful include sickle cell anemia, thalassemia major, severe combined immunodeficiency, chronic granulomatous disease and various malignancies, particularly leukemias and lymphomas.

IMMUNE RESPONSE (IR) GENE

The D sublocus on the HLA locus is involved in both humoral and cell mediated immune responses. Genetics of the mouse indicated that the ability of the immune system to make antibodies to particular antigens is genetically determined. The gene locus for this seems to be linked to the major histocompatibility locus in experimental animals and man. Although the D locus in humans seems to be the most important, patients with ankylosing spondylitis or Reiter's syndrome are usually HLA-B27 histotype.

The major histocompatibility complex in humans occurs on the 6th chromosome. It can be diagrammed as follows.

Association of selected autoimmune diseases with HLA-D locus antigens

Disease	Antigen	Relative Risk
Multiple sclerosis	2	4*
Lupus	3	6
Myasthenia gravis	3	3
Rheumatoid arthritis	4	4

*incidence is 4X other haplotypes

Which of the transplants would be successful?
[answer at bottom of page]

	Donor	Recipient
1.	AA	AB
2.	BB	AB
3.	AB	AA
4.	AB	BB

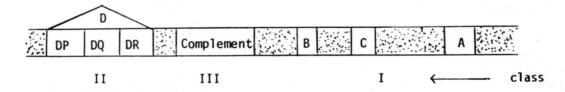

A, B and C = Serologically defined antigens - their presence is detected by cytotoxic of specific antisera plus complement.

D = lymphocyte defined (LD) antigens- antigens detected by mixed lymphocyte reactions. DR, DQ and DP (D related antigens) also code here.

Mixed lymphocyte reaction detects blastogenesis of T lymphocytes in response to histocompatibility antigens foreign on the membrane of the stimulating cell (donor cell: usually a lymphocyte as these cells are particularly rich in these antigens). Donor lymphocytes are poisoned (mitomycin) so they can not divide in response to recipient lymphocytes.

I = genes involved in the recognition and destruction of virally infected activity cells. May also serve as targets in graft rejection.

II = genes involved in immune responses, T & B cell interactions, etc.

III = genes for some of the complement proteins.

[answer to transplant question = 1, 2]

TUMOR IMMUNITY

HUMAN TUMOR IMMUNOLOGY

Some human tumors have characteristic specific antigens, much like the virus induced tumors in animals, such as neuroblastoma and Wilm's tumor, while other tumors have antigens unique to the individual tumor in the individual host (e.g., certain melanoma antigens).

Examples of human tumor-associated antigens (TAAs) include:

1. CEA = carcinoembryonic antigen
2. AFP = alpha fetoprotein
3. PSA = prostate specific antigen
4. M protein = myeloma Igs and fragments such as Bence-Jones
5. Viral antigens such as HBsAg, and Papilloma and Epstein-Barr proteins

There are many malignancies which synthesize embryonic antigens, for example:

Alpha fetoprotein: normally only made by the fetal liver, but also seen in hepatoma, gastric CA, prostate CA. But no all hepatomas make alpha fetoglobulin, so if this were used as a screening test, there would be false negatives.

CEA: a glycoprotein found in the glycocalyx of cells derived from endoderm and present in the GI carcinomas, especially CA of the colon. It is not completely absent in normal individuals. It is used to follow a patient under therapy, as after surgical removal of CA of the colon.

> Tumor specific transplantation antigens (TSTAs) are those against which an immune response could effect irradication of the tumor. They must be expressed on the cell membrane to be accessible to the protective antibodies and regulatory cells of the host. These are the "candidate" vaccines that are being sought.

Tumor Products Which Aid Growth

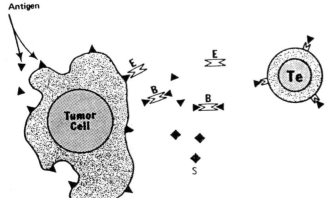

E = Enhancing antibody

B = Blocking factor

S = Suppressor molecules

IMMUNE RESPONSE TO TUMORS

A. __Protective__ to host:

1. Cytotoxic T cells – contact killing – vs tumor antigens.
2. Antibody-dependent cell – mediated cytotoxicity (ADCC) via K cells with receptors for Fc of Ig – contact killing.
3. Natural killer (NK) cells – contact killing.
4. "Activated" macrophages – e.g. via lymphokine (MAF) – "non-specific" contact killing.
5. Cytotoxic antibody (plus complement).

B. __Deleterious__ to host:

1. "Enhancing" antibody – non cytotoxic = combines with tumor target, preventing interaction with cytotoxic T cell.
2. "Blocking" factors, e.g.
   a. Soluble ("Shed") tumor antigen
   b. Antigen (tumor) + antibody complexes combined with cytotoxic T cells or K cells preventing interaction with tumor target.
3. Suppressor (Ts) cells, or their soluble products, interfere with:
   a. cytotoxic T cells
   b. NK cells
   c. antibody (protective) formation

Host Factors Which Limit Tumor Growth

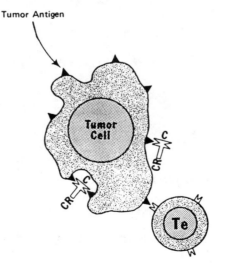

USEFUL TUMOR MARKERS	
Antigen	Cancer
Alpha fetoprotein	Liver, testes
Carcinoembryonic	Colon
Chorionic gonadotropin	Trophoblastic
Immunoglobulin	Myeloma
Acid phosphatase	Prostate
Calcitonin	Thyroid

C = Cytotoxic antibody

CR = Complement receptor

Te = T effector lymphocytes
(cytotoxic cell, etc.)

108

REVIEW STATEMENTS

These should be used to strengthen and expand your understanding of Immunology. If you are uncertain about the veracity of a statement, please "check it out." This will help you strengthen your grasp of the material. You may wish to develop your own list. If you have a spare sheet of paper available, write down the correct statement for every question you miss in going through review exams. This way you can avoid marking on the review exam (so you can use it again) and still have captured that fact for future review.

A graft exchanged between brother and sister is defined as an **allograft**.

Adjuvants are nonspecific, mildly irritating substances which are sometimes used to **enhance antibody responses**.

A graft vs. host reaction occurs when viable immunocompetent cells are put into an immunoincompetent host.

A positive **delayed type hypersensitivity** skin reaction involves a rather complex interaction of antigen, antigen-sensitive lymphocytes and monocytes/macrophages.

Complement activation is involved in production of anaphylotoxins, immune hemolysis, and enhanced phagocytosis.

Lymphokines play an essential role in delayed hypersensitivity reactions.

Examples of cancer-associated antigens which probably arise from tissue de-differentiation include **carcinoembryonic antigen** and **alpha fetoprotein**.

Cell mediated immunity is suppressed by **cortisone**.

A T cell response to basic protein appears to be responsible for the pathogenesis of **experimental allergic encephalomyelitis**.

Leukotriene B4 is chemotactic for neutrophils.

Lymphocytes sensitized to **acetylcholine receptor** appear to be involved in the pathogenesis of **myasthenia gravis**.

Thrombocytopenia, eczema, recurrent pyogenic infections, defective processing of polysaccharide antigens, T-cell deficit, elevated serum IgA, and depressed serum IgM are characteristics of **Wiskott-Aldrich syndrome**.

A serious complication of the use of **immunosuppressive agents** is the increased susceptibility to **opportunistic infections and malignancy**.

IgE attached to basophils and mast cells is essential for **atopic allergy;** allergy and eosinophilia often go hand-in-hand.

Immunodeficiency resulting in susceptibility to **viral infections** is due to a deficiency in T cells.

The target tissues in **Goodpasture's syndrome** are alveolar and glomerular **basement membranes**.

An autoimmune disease with a characteristic IgM antibody response to autologous IgG (g chain) is **rheumatoid arthritis**.

In **systemic lupus erythematosus**, death from renal failure is probably due to glomerular deposition of antigen-antibody-complement complexes.

Anti-thymocyte serum is effective in suppressing allograft rejection because of its ability to suppress cell-mediated immunity.

Chronic graft rejection may be caused by specifically sensitized lymphocytes or humoral antibodies.

Hyperacute graft rejection may be caused by blood group incompatibility between donor and recipient, or previous sensitization of female recipients as a result of multiparity.

A deficiency in **adenosine deaminase** has been observed in many patients with **severe combined immunodeficiency.**

Most **polysaccharide** antigens are **thymus independent** antigens, i.e. they interact directly with B cells to trigger antibody synthesis without the participation of T helper cells and macrophages.

Only **IgG** and **IgM** activate C by the classical pathway.

Clinically, assays for **carcinoembryonic antigen** show their greatest promise in evaluation of completeness of surgical excision of the malignancy, and follow-up for recurrence.

Anaphylatoxin II is a peptide split production of C5 (**C5a**).

Erythroblastosis fetalis is a hemolytic disease in the newborn infant caused by maternal IgG antibody against fetal red cell antigens (usually D).

In humans, **anaphylaxis** results from the combination of allergens with homocytotropic antibodies of the immunoglobulin class **IgE,** which has affinity for mast cells and basophils.

Lesions seen in **serum sickness** result from complexes formed by antigen, complement, and IgG or IgM; the fundamental lesion in immune complex-induced **glomerulonephritis requires neutrophils.**

Immune complexes appear to be involved in the pathogenesis of post-streptococcal glomerulonephritis, the Arthus reaction and glomerulonephritis of systemic lupus erythematosus.

The class of immunoglobulin capable of **passing through the human placenta** from mother to fetus is **IgG.** The **trophoblastic cells** have an **Fcγ receptor** which is essential for this selective transport.

An **Fab fragment** consists of an entire light chain and part of a heavy chain. It is the **antigen-binding fragment;** the antibody paratope is a "mirror image" of the epitope, one of the idiotopes (idiotypes) is the paratope.

Erythroblastosis fetalis can be prevented if the mother is injected, at parturition, with a monomeric anti-Rh^O antibody called **Rhogam.**

Specific immunologic tolerance is most easily induced in T cells.

The complement components which react in the classical pathway but not in the C3 bypass are C1, C4 and C2.

Individuals with **hereditary angioneurotic edema** have a deficiency in **C1 esterase inhibitor**.

Innate immunity can be defined as a complex, naturally-occurring system of defense mechanisms which protect the individual from infectious agents.

Interferon induces cells to produce anti-viral proteins which **interfer with translation of viral mRNA.**

Heptamer-nonamer base pairing in introns between V, J, and D regions bring the exons into juxtaposition to allow **recombinase enzymes** to effect the genetic recombination necessary to assemble immunoglobulin molecules. **Looping out of extraneous RNA and RNA splicing** occurs after transcription and is the final step in the synthesis of H and L chain mRNA; it joins the constant region gene product to the rest of the mRNA.

The **membrane attack complex** consists of complement components C5 - 9; the late molecules are **like porins**, they intercalate, polymerize, and form pores in the membrane - thus the cell lyses.

The rapid rise, elevated level, and prolonged production of antibody which follows a second exposure to antigen is called **anamnesis**, and is mainly IgG.

Complement is involved in Gell and Coombs **type II and III hypersensitivities**, not in types I or IV.

Mature B cells have surface immunoglobulin of the **IgM** and **IgD** classes.

IgM is the major antibody that **a fetus** can make; if level is elevated at birth it may signify **fetal infection**.

The thymus and the bone marrow are the **primary lymphoid organs** of mammals and are the sites of T and B cell maturation, rerspectively.

Mu and epsilon heavy chains have **5 domains**; gamma and alpha heavy chains have 4; all light chains have 2 domains (1 variable and 1 constant).

The radioallergosorbent test (**RAST**) measures IgG specific for a given allergen, while the paper radioimmunosorbent test (**PRIST**) quantitates the total serum IgE.

Aryl sulfatase, an enzyme of eosinophil origin, **inactivates SRS-A,** slow reacting substance of anaphylaxis.

The **IgG blocking antibodies** which are produced after allergen injection protect the allergic individual by **competing with cell-bound IgE** for the triggering antigen.

The **most common immunoglobulin deficiency** disease involves absence of **IgA**.

Patients with **deficiencies of C5-9** have an increased occurrence and severity of infections caused by **gonococci** and the **meningococci.**

Leukotrienes **C4, D4** and **E4** effect smooth muscles and **increase vascular permeability.**

T cells undergo blastogenesis when they interact with their homologous epitope.

Most **interleukins** are produced by T cells; their targets are usually other cells of the immune system, either T or B cells. They may also activate macrophages or NK cells and have stimulatory activity on other cells of the body; they **are promiscuous cell stimulants.**

IL-1 is produced by macrophages and activates various cells of the body, primarily T helper cells and B cells. It is also an autocrine (stimulates other macrophages) and causes pyrexia (**endogenous pyrogen**).

IL-2 is a T cell product which induces proliferation and maturation of both B and T cells.

IL-4 is a T cell product that enhances **class switching** in B cells; it favors IgG1 and IgE production.

IL-6 is a T cell product that enhances B cell proliferation and immunoglobulin secretion in B cells.

IL-10 is a Th2 cell product that inhibits cytokine production (e.g., Il-2, Il-4, IFN-γ) by Th1 cells.

Interferon gamma has antiviral activity; it also induces the expression of MHC class II molecules on tissue cells and activates macrophages and NK cells. It is produced by T cells.

Lectins are proteins (usually from plants) that bind to sugar residues in membranes of mammalian cells.

Antibody diversity is due to 1) presence of **multiple V, J and D region genes,** 2) **random assortment** of H and L chains, 3) **junctional and insertional imprecision**, and 4) **somatic cell mutations.**

Allelic exclusion is the ability of B cells **to product a single H and a single L chain** and exclude the second set of genes on the other chromosome. This process ensures that both valences on the antibody react with the same epitope.

Langerhans cells in the skin are effective **antigen presenting** cells, particularly in DTH reactions.

Cytotoxic T cells (and NK cells) **are NOT destroyed** in the process of killing other cells.

Alternative complement pathway is an antibody INdependent complement activation system involving C3-C9 and factors B, D, H, I and P.

Antibody-dependent cell mediated cytotoxicity (ADCC) is a type of cell-mediated cytotoxic reaction in which a target cell with bound antibody is recognized by an effector cell bearing Fc receptors and is subsequently lysed without complement involvement.

Bence-Jones proteins are monoclonal immunoglobulin light chains present (usually as dimers) in the urine of some patients with multiple myeloma.

CD2 is a glycoprotein expressed on most thymocytes, all peripheral T cells, and on large granular lymphocytes. The molecule serves as a signal transducing molecule and as a cell-adhesion molecule.

CD3 is a complex of 5 polypeptides associated with the T-cell receptor; it serves as a signal transducing molecule and as a cell adhesion molecule.

CD4 is a cell surface glycoprotein found on the subset of T cells (usually T_H) that recognizes antigenic peptides "presented" in the groove of the class II MHC.

CD8 is a cell surface glycoprotein found on the subset of T cells (usually T_C) that recognizes antigenic peptides presented in the groove of a class I MHC molecules.

The **class I MHC** molecule is composed of an integral membrane polypeptide noncovalently associated with β-2 microglobulin and **found on all nucleated cells** of the body. Class I MHC is encoded by HLA-A, B, and C in humans.

The **Class II MHC** molecule consists of two integral membrane polypeptides encoded by HLA-DR, DQ, and DP in humans. These molecules are expressed on **macrophages, B cells, dendritic cells,** and **other antigen-presenting cells.**

Class III MHC gene products of a MHC region are distinct from class I and class II MHC molecules, and include some components of the complement system, steroid 21-hydroxylase enzymes, and TNF α and β.

Clonal selection is a central theory of immunology in which antigen binds to and stimulates a particular lymphocyte to undergo mitosis and develop into a clone of cells with identical immunologic specificity.

Cytokines are a group of small proteins that regulate the intensity of an immune response by stimulating or inhibiting the proliferation and/or secretory activity of various immune cells.

Delayed type hypersensitivity (DTH) is a type IV hypersensitive response mediated by sensitized T lymphocytes. The response is characterized by the recruitment and activation of macrophages. The response generally occurs within 48-72 hrs and manifests as chronic inflammatiory lesions, granuloma formation, tuberculin reactivity, and contact hypersensitivity.

DiGeorge syndrome is a congenital immunodeficiency syndrome characterized by the absence of a thymus, hypoparathyroidism, and cardiovascular anomalies. The absence of a thymus results in the absence of cell-mediated immunity.

The **Fab fragment** is a monovalent antigen-binding fragment of an immunoglobulin obtained by **papain** digestion that is composed of the light chain and part of the heavy chain.

The **F(ab')$_2$ fragment** is a bivalent antigen-binding fragment of an immunoglobulin obtained by **pepsin** digestion that contains both light chains and part of both heavy chains.

Fc fragment is the crystallizable, non-antigen binding portion of an immunoglobulin molecule derived from digestion with **papain.** It contains the binding sites for Fc receptors and the C1q component of complement.

Fc receptor is a cellular membrane componment that is specific for the Fc portion of certain classes of immunoglobulin.

112

A **hybridoma** is a cell line derived by fusion of a lymphocyte and a tumor cell. The resulting hybridoma continues to secrete the antibody of the normal B cell but retains the immortal growth properties of the myeloma cell.

Hypervariable regions are amino acid sequences within the variable regions of heavy and light immunoglobulin chains and of the T cell receptor that contribute most to the antigen-binding site. Synonymous with complementarity determining regions (CDRs).

Framework regions are relatively conserved sequences of amino acids located on either side of the CDRs in heavy and light chain variable regions of immunoglobulin. These conserved sequences generate the beta pleated sheet structure of the V_H and V_L domains.

Immunoglobulin superfamily proteins contain domains such as those found in immunoglobulins, the T-cell receptor and MHC membrane molecules.The domains are formed by intrachain disulfide linkages.

Intron are noncoding gene segments which separate **exons or coding regions**. Introns are initially transcribed in the primary transcript but are removed by RNA splicing during formation of mRNA.

Exon is any continous seqment of a gene whose sequence can be found in the mature RNA product of that gene. Most genes are composed of 2 or more exons separated from one another by introns.

Interferons (IFN) are a family of glycoproteins that induce an antiviral state in cells and help to regulate the immune response. IFN-α is derived from various leukocytes, IFN-β is derived from fibroblasts and IFN-γ is produced by T lymphocytes.

NK (natural killer) cells are large, granular lymphoid cells bearing Fc receptors that destroy target cells by ADCC. They destroy some tumor cells without MHC restriction.

Langerhans cells are a type of dendritic cell found in the skin that serve as an antigen-presenting cell.

Leukocyte functional antigens (LFA-1, LFA-2, and LFA-3) mediate intercellular adhesion.

Leukotrienes are mediators of type I hypersensitivity formed by the mast cell or blood basophil. They are metabolic products of arachidonic acid produced by the lipoxygenase pathway.

Lymphokine activated killer cells are NK cells that have been activated by IL-2 and exhibit more effective killing of their target cells.

Lymphotoxin (LT) is produced by activated T cells.

The membrane attack complex (MAC) consists of complement components C5-C9 that create a polyperforin pore in target cells.

MHC restriction is the requirement that T cells recognize antigen only when antigenic peptides are displayed in association with self MHC molecules.

An **Opsonin** is a substance, such as an antibody or C3b, which binds to an antigen and enhances phagocytosis.

PAF (Platelet activating factor) is released by basophils and mast cells during a type I hypersensitivity reaction; it causes aggregation and lysis of platelets with release of histamine.

Paratope is an idiotope of an antibody or a T-cell receptor that is directly involved in binding to the epitope of an antigen.

Second-set graft rejection is an acute, rapid rejection of an allograft in an individual immunized by a previous graft. It is an anamnestic response to the graft.

Serum sickness is a type III hypersensitivity reaction that develops when antigen is administered intravenously, resulting in large amounts of antigen-antibody complexes. The deposition of the immune complexes leads to vasculitis, glomerulonephritis, and arthritis. Serum sickness often develops when individuals are immunized with antiserum derived from another species (e.g. horse anti-venin).

113

Slow-reacting substances of anaphylaxis (SRS-A) are leukotrienes formed by mast cells and basophils which cause smooth muscle contraction.

Northern Blot is a technique for detection of specific **RNA species** within a complex mixture of **RNAs** after separation by gel electrophoresis.

Southern blot technique uses electrophoretic separation of **DNA fragments,** transfer or blotting of ssDNA to a suitable filter, and hybridization of the separated ssDNA fragments with a complementary radioactive nucleic acid probe.

Western blot involves detection of **protein antigens** that have been electrophoretically seperated and transferred to a filter such as nitrocellulose by labeling the antigenic bands with radioactive or enzyme-conjugated antibodies.

Addressins are surface macromolecules on endothelial cells that serve as homing receptors for circulating lymphocytes.

Selectins are proteins that have lectinlike oligosaccharide-binding activity, and function in cell "homing".

Am marker is the allotoypic determinant on the heavy chain of human IgA.

Gm marker is the allotypic determinant on the heavy chain of human IgG.

Km marker is the allotypic determinant on the human kappa light chain.

C-myc gene is a member of a candidate set of cancer-related genes or cellular oncogenes. **C-myc** protein is thought to be involved in regulating cell proliferation. Abnormal expression of c-Myc contributes to development of certain cancers, including Burkitt's lymphoma.

Cold agglutinins are antibodies that agglutinate better at temperatures below 37 $^\circ$C than at 37°C.

CREST phenomenon is phenomenon that consists of calcinosis, Raynaud's phenomenon, esophageal dysmotility, sclerodactyly, and telangiectasis. The patients have antibodies to the centromere.

Defensins are antimicrobial peptides found in neutrophil granules.

Counter immunoelectrophoresis is an immunodiffusion technique in which antigen and antibody are driven toward each other in an electrical field and then precipitate.

Molecular mimicry is the immunologic cross-reactivity shared between determinants on an environmental antigen (such as a bacterium) and a self antigen; this relatedness has been proposed to explain autoimmunity.

Myeloma proteins are monoclonal immunoglobulin molecules, or a portion thereof, that are produced by malignant plasma cells.

Pre-B cells are B lymphocyte precursors found predominantly in the bone marrow and characterized by the presence of cytoplasmic immunoglobulin heavy chains without surface immunoglobulins.

Recombinases are enzymes that carries out V/D/J exon rearrangements.

Superantigens are a group of bacterial or viral proteins that activate T cells bearing a specific class of Vβ chain; they are polyclonal activators.

The T$_H$1 lymphocyte is a helper T cell that elaborates cytokines (such as IFNγ) which selectively promote **cell-mediated immune responses**.

T$_H$2 lymphocyte is a helper T cell that elaborates cytokines (including IL-4, IL-5, IL-6, and IL-10) which selectively promote **humoral immune responses**.

Transgenic refers to an organism (usually multicellular) into whose genome a foreign gene has been introduced.

IMMUNOLOGY REVIEW EXAM

SELECT THE SINGLE BEST COMPLETION FOR EACH QUESTION BELOW.

1. Patients with Bruton's disease may fail to produce IgG in response to immunization with diphtheria toxoid because they

    A. have a decreased number of B cells.
    B. have an increased number of T suppressor cells.
    C. lack CD4+ T helper cells.
    D. have a faulty antigen processing macrophage.
    E. have a faulty class switching mechanism.

2. A mutation in the heptamer-nonamer sequences in germline immunoglobulin DNA would probably prevent

    A. cleavage of leader sequences.
    B. isotype switching.
    C. V to J rearrangement and joining.
    D. RNA splicing.

3. Antibody to acetylcholine receptors is found in patients with

    A. Multiple sclerosis.
    B. Muscular dystrophy.
    C. Myasthenia gravis.
    D. Graves' disease.
    E. Pernicious anemia.

4. Which of the following immune deficiency disorders is associated exclusively with an abnormality of C1 esterase activity ?

    A. Bruton's disease
    B. DiGeorge syndrome
    C. Wiskoff-Aldrich syndrome
    D. Chronic mucocutaneous candidiasis
    E. Hereditary angioneurotic edema

5. Blocking factors formed during tumor growth

    A. bind to T lymphocytes and induce lysis of tumor cells.
    B. block the stimulation of tumor-specific B cells.
    C. block growth of tumor cells.
    D. block the action of cytotoxic T lymphocytes on tumor cells.
    E. activate complement and cause tumor cell lysis.

6. Synovial fluid of patients with rheumatoid arthritis is likely to contain an IgM antibody reactive with

    A. light chain determinants of IgG.
    B. heavy chain determinants of IgG.
    C. cross reacting bacterial antigens.
    D. synovial cell membranes.
    E. J chain determinants of IgA.

7. Immunotoxins are

    A. monokines released by macrophages.
    B. toxins coupled to antigen-specific immunoglobulins.
    C. toxins complexed with homologous antitoxins.
    D. lymphokines.
    E. lymphotoxins.

8. Tetanus neonatorum kills hundreds of thousands of children in third world countries each year. The best way to provide immunologic protection is to

A. inject the infant with human tetanus antitoxin.
B. inject the newborn with tetanus toxoid.
C. inject the mother with antitoxin 72 hours before the birth of her child.
D. immunize the mother with tetanus toxoid early in pregnancy.
E. give the child antitoxin and toxoid for both passive and active immunization.

9. Which of the following antibody iso-types can cause erythroblastosis fetalis?

A. IgG
B. IgM
C. IgA
D. IgE
E IgG and IgM

10. The CD4 molecule

A. differs in amino acid sequence on cells with different antigen-specificity.
B. is the receptor for sheep erythrocytes.
C. is the receptor which recognizes antigen.
D. plays a role in the recognition of MHC class II molecules.
E. plays a role in the recognition of MHC class I molecules.

11. Natural isohemagglutinins are

A. IgG antibodies which are produced without any prior antigenic stimulation.
B. IgM antibodies which are produced without any prior antigenic stimulation.
C. able to cross the placenta.
D. the most likely cause of transfusion reactions resulting from ABO incompatibility.

12. The CD3 molecule

A. differs in amino acid sequence on cells with different antigen-specificity.
B. is the receptor for sheep erythrocytes.
C. is closely linked to the receptor that recognizes antigen.
D. plays a role in the recognition of MHC class II molecules.
E. plays a role in the recognition of MHC class I molecules.

13. A pre-B cell generally expresses

A. both cytoplasmic and membrane-bound μ chains and MHC class II molecules.
B. cytoplasmic μ chains and MHC class II molecules.
C. cytoplasmic μ chains but not MHC class I molecules.
D. membrane (surface) IgM and IgD.
E. CD3.

14. Under which of the following conditions do graft-versus host (GVH) reactions occur ?

A. When the graft is contaminated with gram-negative microorganisms
B. When tumor tissues are grafted
C. When viable T cells are present in the graft
D. When the graft has histocom-patibility antigens not found in the recipient
E. When the graft is pretreated with antilymphocyte serum

15. Efficient T-cell mediated killing of virus infected cells requires major histocom-patibility complex (MHC) antigen compatibility with

A. ABO blood group antigens.
B. Rh blood group antigens.
C. class I antigens.
D. class II antigens.
E. class III antigens.

16. Induction of blocking antibodies by injection of allergen

    A. is safe if used initially with high concentrations of antigen.
    B. should be done by a trained health care provider that has epinephrine available in case of an adverse reaction.
    C. directly affects stability of membranes.
    D. is a form of passive immunity.
    E. induces large amounts of endogenous antihistamines.

17. A 6 year old male was hospitalized for bacterial meningitis. Cultures of sputum and CSF yielded many colonies of *Haemophilus influenzae*. Past history indicated that the patient had numerous bacterial infections including seven episodes of pneumonia. Physical exam showed that tonsillar tissue was scanty. A lymph node biopsy revealed that germinal centers were absent, but that paracortical and medullary areas had normal numbers of lymphocytes. A mumps skin test was positive. Additional studies on this patient would probably show

    A. a normal *in vitro* response to PHA.
    B. absence of circulating B cells.
    C. very low (less than 200 mg/dl) serum immunoglobulin levels.
    D. a positive mumps C fixation test.

18. Rebecca, a seven month old child was hospitalized for a yeast infection that would not respond to therapy. The patient had a history of acute pyogenic infections. Physical examination revealed that the spleen and lymph nodes were not palpable. The patient is extremely lymphopenic. This history is compatible with

    A. chronic mucocutaneous candidiasis.
    B. Wiscott-Aldrich syndrome.
    C. X-linked agammaglobulinemia.
    D. severe combined immuno-deficiency disease.

19. Which of the following are markers of mature B cells?

    A. Receptors that react with CD3 molecules.
    B. Membrane-associated CD3 molecules.
    C. Unrearranged germline configuration of genes for H chains.
    D. Membrane associated IgM and IgD.

20. A 7-month-old girl who has a history of pyogenic infections is hospitalized with *Candida albicans* pharyngitis. A differential white blood cell count shows 95% neutrophils, 1% lymphocytes and 48% monocytes. X-ray reveals absence of a thymic shadow. These findings are most compatible with

    A. multiple myeloma
    B. severe combined immunodeficiency disease
    C. x-linked agammaglobulinemia
    D. Wiskott-Aldrich syndrome
    E. chronic granulomatous disease

21. Which of the following disorders is an autoimmune disease with a characteristic antibody response to autologous IgG?

    A. Pernicious anemia
    B. Rheumatoid arthritis
    C. Goodpasture's syndrome
    D. Myasthenia gravis
    E. Wiskott-Aldrich syndrome

22. You prescribe penicillin for your patient. The patient develops a severe allergic reaction and dies. in this case, the penicillin molecule was probably acting as a (an)

    A. adjuvant.
    B. hapten.
    C. immunologic carrier.
    D. immunotoxin.

117

23. The class-specific antigenic determinants of immunoglobulins are associated with

 A. framework residues of variable regions of both and heavy and light chains.
 B. constant regions of the light chain.
 C. constant regions of the heavy chain.
 D. variable regions of the light chain.
 E. variable regions of the heavy chain.

24. Serum obtained from a 32 week human fetus would probably contain

 A. maternal IgM and fetal IgG antibodies.
 B. maternal IgG and fetal IgM antibodies.
 C. maternal IgG antibodies only.
 D. fetal IgM antibodies only.

25. In the context of immunoglobulin synthesis, allelic exclusion is essential in order to insure that

 A. leader sequences are removed by a post-translational cleavage.
 B. antibodies have the desired immunologic specificity.
 C. antibodies have a wide range of distinct biological activities.
 D. antibodies are functionally divalent.

26. If you could analyze, at the molecular level, a plasma cell that is making IgG antibody, you would find the following:

 A. a DNA sequence for VD and J genes translocated near the gamma-DNA exon.
 B. mRNA specific for both the kappa and lambda light chains.
 C. mRNA specific for J chains.
 D. DNA sequence for VD and J genes translocated near the kappa-DNA exon.
 E. the c-myc gene translocated near the gamma-DNA exon.

27. Properdin has the effect of amplifying complement activation by

 A. facilitating the binding of Factor B to C3b.
 B. facilitating the binding of Factor D to C3b.
 C. stabilization of the C3bBb complex.
 D. promoting the binding of C1q to antibody.
 E. facilitating binding of the membrane attack complex (C5-9) to the cell.

28. VDJ immunoglobulin gene rearrangement

 A. occurs prior to exposure of the B cell to antigen.
 B. is induced in B cells by antigen.
 C. can occur either prior to or subsequent to exposure to antigen.
 D. occurs only after the immunoglobulin light chain genes have undergone rearrangement.

29. Interferon causes antiviral resistance by inducing intracellular formation of antiviral proteins that

 A. interfere with adsorption of viruses to other cells
 B. prevent penetration of viruses
 C. block transcription of viral nucleic acid
 D. block translation of viral nucleic acid

30. An idiotype is

 A. determined by the amino acid residues in the framework regions.
 B. determined by the amino acid residues in the hypervariable regions.
 C. often expressed on CD4 or CD8 molecules.
 D. expressed only after a B cell has been exposed to antigen.

31. The compound receptor characteristic of Th cells consists of T cell receptor and CD4 which recognize processed antigen and

    A. CD3.
    B. antibody.
    C. classI MHC.
    D. class II MHC.

32. Three weeks following an influenza vaccine shot, a 46-year-old pathologist has progressive weakness in his arms and legs He begins to have difficulty breathing and is brought to the hospital. On physical examination, absence of deep tendon reflexes is noted. The most likely diagnosis is

    A. influenza.
    B. Guillain-Barre' syndrome.
    C. Creutzfeldt - Jakob.
    D. muscular dystrophy.
    E. myasthenia gravis.

33. Which one of the following substances works to directly reverse bronchoconstriction and hence is the treatment of choice in severe allergic respiratory distress?

    A. Cromolyn sodium
    B. Antihistamines
    C. Epinephrine
    D. Blocking antibody

34. Which of the following drugs blocks release of mediators from mast cells?

    A. Cromolyn sodium
    B. Antihistamines
    C. Epinephrine
    D. Blocking antibody

35. Which of the following substances could prevent ragweed allergen from reaching sensitized mast cells?

    A. Cromolyn sodium
    B. IgG anti-ragweed antibodies
    C. Epinephrine
    D. Antihistamines

36. Positive skin tests to *Candida albicans* or tuberculoprotein have certain aspects in common with a reaction to poison ivy. These similarities include the following:

    A. They both are chemical responses to caustic irritants.
    B. They both are due to IgE antibody.
    C. They both occur within 1 hour of antigen exposure.
    D. They both are T cell-mediated.

37. Gel electrophoresis is used to separate mixtures of antigens. Serum can then be analyzed for epitope-specific antibodies by a procedure called

    A. Immunoelectrophoresis
    B. Western blotting
    C. Radioimmunoassay
    D. Counter Immunoelectro-phoresis
    E. Enzyme linked immuno-sorbent assays

38. The results of a blood test for HIV-1 for one of your patients indicate that antibodies are detectable by ELISA using plates coated with HIV-1 lysates. However, Western blots are negative for HIV-1. The most likely interpretation of these data is that

    A. lab tech doesn't know how to perform a Western blot.
    B. patient is infected with HIV-2.
    C. ELISA data represent a false positive reaction.
    D. Western blot data represent a false negative reaction.

39. Class I restriction refers to

    A. T cell - B cell interaction.
    B. T cell - antigen processing cell interaction.
    C. antibody formation.
    D. Tc - target cell recognition.

119

40. A 4-year old child suffering from repeated pyogenic infections was found to have normal phagocytic function and cell mediated immune responses. Lymph node biopsy would probably reveal

A. depletion of thymus-dependent regions
B. intact germinal centers
C. absence of dendritic cells
D. paucity of plasma cells

41. Your 3-year-old patient received the standard DPT immunization series starting at 3 months of age, however he has no detectable antibody to diphtheria, pertussis, or tetanus. You are faced with treating him for a deep puncture wound. The best treatment to prevent tetanus would be an injection of

A. tetanus toxoid.
B. tetanus bacilli plus toxoid.
C. tetanus antitoxin (equine).
D. tetanus immune globulin (human).
E. lymphocytes from a hyperimmunized veterinarian.

42. IgG molecules preferentially cross the human placenta because the

A. IgG antibody is the major immunoglobulin in the mother's circulation.
B. the trophoblastic cells have FcgR in their membranes.
C. this immunoglobulin is the major source of passive immunity for the infant.
D. the uterus has high levels of IgG-producing plasma cells.
E. the placenta has high levels of IgG-producing plasma cells.

43. Infantile X-linked agammaglobulinemia occurs in male infants, who begin to suffer from recurrent bacterial infections at about 9-12 months of age. Patients have no plasma cells; their blood lymphocytes lack surface immunoglobulins. Which of the following is true ?

A. The age of onset of infections is due to disappearance of maternal antibody
B. The disease is most easily diagnosed by measuring CD4+ lymphocytes in the patient's peripheral blood
C. The defect may be in stem cell differentiation, as indicated by the occurrence of global immunodeficiency
D. the B cell response is intact, but the defect is in antigen processing

44. A patient who is allergic to ragweed developed IgE myeloma. The myeloma IgE does not react with the ragweed pollen. What would be the effect of his myeloma on the severity of his allergic symptoms during hay fever season?

A. No change
B. Increase due to his having more IgE
C. Increase due to the blocking effect of the myeloma
D. Decrease due to the displacement of IgE anti-ragweed on mast cell by myeloma IgE

45. In the direct immunofluorescence identification of *Treponema pallidum* fluorescein is conjugated to

A. the microorganism
B. C3b
C. antibody specific to human gamma globulin
D. antibody specific to the microorganism
E. antibody specific to complement

46. After a bone marrow transplant from his HLA matched sister, Jimmy developed a syndrome characterized by pancytopenia, aplastic anemia, skin rash, diarrhea, jaundice and weight loss. This condition is called

A. allograft rejection
B. graft versus host disease
C. failure of bone marrow engraftment
D. a secondary infection
E. anamnesis

47. A young boy has had repeated infections with *Staphylococcus aureus*. His laboratory data reveals that he has normal numbers of white blood cells with a normal distribution by differential counting. His immunoglobulin levels are normal and he responds to candida skin test antigen with a positive DTH reaction. Which of the following types of immune deficiency do you suspect?

A. T cell deficiency
B. B cell deficiency
C. Granulocyte disorder
D. Combined immunodeficiency

48. The basis for the control which MHC molecules have over the immune response is best explained by the

A. ability of MHC-antigen complexes to be released from antigen processing cells and stimulate the activation of lymphocytes
B. expression of MHC gene products on effector T and B lymphocytes
C. existence of genes controlling the immune response in linkage disequilibrium with MHC genes
D. need for antigen-derived peptides to bind an MHC class I or class II molecule for proper presentation to the receptor of a T lymphocyte
E. special affinity of unprocessed antigens for MHC molecules

49. A recipient of a 2-haplotype (i.e. both chromosomes) MHC-matched kidney from a relative still needs immunosuppression to prevent graft rejection because

A. graft-versus-host disease is a problem
B. class II MHC antigens will not be matched
C. minor histocompatibility antigens will not be matched
D. immunosuppression decreases the chance of infection at the surgical site

50. The activated macrophage kills tumor cells by secretion of

A. GM-CSF
B. reactive nitrogen intermediates
C. perforins
D. IL-10
E. IL-12

51. Epinephrine is valuable in the management of atopy through its ability to block mediator release by

A. inhibiting phosphodiesterase
B. inhibiting production of histamine
C. inhibiting slow-reacting substance of anaphylaxis (SRS-A)
D. stimulating adenylate cyclase
E. stimulating release of lymphokines

52. All of the following are clinical expressions of a humoral immune response **EXCEPT**

    A. Atopic dermatitis
    B. Poststreptococcal glomerulonephritis
    C. Hemolytic disease of the newborn
    D. Food allergy
    E. Contact dermatitis

53. Which of the following is **NOT** an assay of B cell competence ?

    A. Serum immunoglobulin levels
    B. Isohemagglutinin titers
    C. Chemotaxis
    D. Assay for lymphocytes bearing surface IgM
    E. Assay for lymphocytes bearing antibody and complement receptors

54. General signs of autoimmune disease which may be of diagnostic importance include all of the following **EXCEPT**

    A. depressed serum gamma globulin levels.
    B. depressed serum complement levels.
    C. increased immune complexes in serum.
    D. presence of autoantibodies in serum.
    E. depressed levels of Ts cells in peripheral blood.

55. Hemolytic anemia may result from all of the following **EXCEPT**

    A. passive transfer of maternal Rh antibody to the fetus.
    B. transfusion of autologous cryopreserved red cells.
    C. production of antibody to certain drugs.
    D. production of cold agglutinins after certain viral infections.

56. The administration of vaccines is not without hazard. Of the following, which is **LEAST** likely to adversely affect an immunocompromised host ?

    A. Measles vaccine
    B. Hepatitis B vaccine
    C. Rubella vaccine
    D. Mumps vaccine
    E. Sabin poliomyelitis vaccine

57. Activation of the alternative pathway of complement can involve all of the following **EXCEPT**

    A. utilization of properdin.
    B. utilization of C3.
    C. formation of C3bBb.
    D. utilization of C2.
    E. utilization of the membrane attack complex.

58. Preformed (in the mast cell) mediators of anaphylaxis include all of the following **EXCEPT**

    A. histamine.
    B. eosinophil chemotactic factor of anaphylaxis.
    C. heparin.
    D. serotonin.
    E. slow reacting substance of anaphylaxis.

59. Antimicrobial factors that are a part of the first line of defense include all of the following **EXCEPT**

    A. fatty acids from sebaceous glands.
    B. antibodies in saliva.
    C. lysozyme in tears.
    D. acid in gastric juices.
    E. Kupffer cells in the liver.

60. All of the following are true of anti-idiotype antibodies **EXCEPT**

    A. mimic the antigenic epitope.
    B. bind with the paratope of the antibody reactive with the epitope that elicited the original (first) antibody.
    C. regulate the immune response.
    D. bind to T cell receptors for antigen.
    E. induce immune tolerance.

61. Antibody diversity is generated by all of the following **EXCEPT**

    A. J chain association with mu heavy chains.
    B. combinatorial association of different V and J exons.
    C. flexible recombination (V and J exons can join at slightly different sites).
    D. somatic mutation.
    E. random assortment of heavy and light chains.

62. Which of the following is **NOT** true of the thymus ?

    A. A lymphoid organ where extensive cell proliferation and cell death occur.
    B. The organ where T lymphocytes acquire antigen-specific receptors.
    C. The organ where T cells acquire markers enabling them to leave the circulation.
    D. An organ that is maximally active early in life.
    E. A primary site of antibody synthesis.

63. Helper T cells can induce all of the following **EXCEPT**

    A. proliferation of B cells.
    B. differentiation of B cells into plasma cells.
    C. expansion of the pool of memory B cells.
    D. immunoglobulin class switching.
    E. graft versus host disease.

64. All of the following immunosuppressive drugs poison rapidly proliferating cells **EXCEPT**

    A. azathioprine.
    B. 6-mercaptopurine.
    C. cyclosporin.
    D. cyclophosphamide.
    E. methotrexate.

65. Activation of the complement cascade plays an important role in host defense by all of the following **EXCEPT**

    A. working via the classical pathway, together with antibody, to induce bacteriolysis.
    B. mediating bacteriolysis directly, via the alternative pathway, in the absence of specific antibody.
    C. facilitating phagocytosis by generating opsonins.
    D. attracting phagocytes to the site of an infection by generating chemotaxins.
    E. enhancing the generation of toxic oxygen metabolites during HMP shunt glycolysis.

66. A secondary immune response differs from a primary immune response in each of the following **EXCEPT**

    A. length of the latent period.
    B. higher concentration of antibody activity .
    C. duration of the steady state.
    D. idiotypic specificity.
    E. predominant immunoglobulin class.

67. In general, three types of cells (Th cells, B cells, and antigen presenting cells) collaborate in the induction of a humoral immune response. Which of these cell types **DOES NOT** exhibit immunologic specificity?

    A. Th cells
    B. B cells
    C. Antigen presenting cells
    D. Th and antigen presenting cells
    E. Th and B cells

68. The major histocompatibility complex (MHC) of humans (i.e. the HLA) is composed of linked genetic loci whose collective products are characterized by all of the following **EXCEPT**

A. class I, class II, and class III antigens and b2-microglobulin are included.
B. some are strong barriers to tissue transplantation.
C. some are complement components.
D. some are necessary for interactions among antigen processing cells, T cells and B cells.
E. their cellular and/or humoral distribution is diverse.

69. Clinical findings in a patient with lupus may include all of the following **EXCEPT**

A. malar rash.
B. oral ulcers.
C. serositis.
D. psychoses.
E. Osler's nodes.

70. Tommy presents to your office with otitis media; you prescribe penicillin per os. That evening Tommy develops a rash and begins to experience respiratory difficulty. Which of the following would be the **BEST** therapy at this time?

A. administer epinephrine
B. nebulize the patient with cromolyn sodium
C. switch antibiotics and give the paitient cephalothin.
D. add dexamethasone to the therapy.
E. give the patient benedryl

DIRECTIONS (Items 71-96): Each set of matching questions in this section consists of a list of up to 26 lettered options, followed by several numbered items. For each numbered item, select the ONE lettered option that is most closely associated with it. An answer may be used once, more than once, or not at all.

Match the region of the immunoglobulin molecule with the description that applies.

A. Constant region of the light chain

B. Hypervariable regions

C. Light chain

D. J region

E. Constant regions of the heavy chain

F. Fd fragment

G. D region

H. Hinge region

71. The portion of an immunoglobulin molecule that determines its biological activity

72. The portion of an immunoglobulin molecule that determines its isotype

73. The portion of an immunoglobulin molecule that is recognized by anti-idiotypic antibody

74. The portion of an immunoglobulin molecule that binds to antigen

A.	Th lymphocyte	F.	Eosinophil
B.	B lymphocyte	G.	Neutrophil
C.	Macrophage	H.	Langerhans cell
D.	Natural Killer cells	I.	Ts lymphocyte
E.	Mast cell	J.	Tc lymphocyte

75.   Source of mediators in Hay fever

76.   Important in antibody dependent cellular cytotoxicity

77.   Major role in immune surveillence

78.   CD4+ inducer cell for delayed type hypersensitivity

For each patient, select the phrase that best matches each immunologic disorder.

A.	Delayed hypersensitivity to myelin	F.	Type I hypersensitivity to myelin
B.	Autoimmune disease of peripheral nervous system	G.	Autoantibodies to g heavy chains
		H.	Autoantibodies to centromeres
C.	Immune complex deposition in skin	I.	Autoantibodies to islet cells in pancreas
D.	Autoantibodies to the acetylcholine receptor	J.	Antithyroglobulin autoantibodies
E.	Autoantibodies to TSH		

79.   A 37 year old school nurse presents with arthritis, pleuritis, and low grade fever. She has anti ds DNA antibodies in her serum. The symptoms began shortly after she began taking hydralazine to control her hypertension.

80.   This 33 hear old clinical psychologist has lost 18 pounds despite his robust eating habits. He reports cardiac palpitation and moderate dysphagia; the latter appears to be due to hyperplasia of the thyroid.

81.   A 13 year old boy scout presents with symptoms of anorexia, nausea and abdominal pain. He reports frequent need to urinate. His blood glucose is very high; bicarbonate and pCO_2 are low.

82.   A patient presents with calcinosis, Raynaud's phenomenon, esophageal dysmotility, sclerodactyly and telangiectases.

83.   A 57 year old Dentist develops generalized malaise and muscular weakness two weeks after a serious bout of influenza. This condition worsens over the next 6 days and he is admitted to the hospital when his extremities become so weak he is unable to get out of bed. During the ensuring 3 weeks his conditions continued to deteriorate and his paralysis became almost complete.

A.	Alpha Fetoprotein	E.	Calcitonin
B.	Carcinoembryonic Antigen	F.	Epstein-Barr glycoprotein
C.	CALLA	G.	Cardiolipin
D.	Bence Jones protein	H.	HIVgp120

84.   Primary carcinoma of the liver

85.   Multiple myeloma

86.   Colorectal carcinoma

A.	Pooled gamma globulin (human)	G.	Killed virus vaccine and
B.	Specific immune globulin		specific immune globulin
	(human)		(human)
C.	Transfusion of erythrocytes	H.	Live virus vaccine
D.	Bone marrow transplant	I.	Specific immune globulin
E.	Fetal thymus transplant		(horse)
F.	Toxoid and specific immune	J.	Transfusion of neutrophils
	globulin (human)		

87.   One year old infant who has chronic thrush infection. No problems with other infectious agents are
       reported.

88.   Diminutive 6 year old boy who has had repeated pulmonary infections with normally non-
       pathogenic agents. He had a normal recovery from chickenpox at the age of 34 months.

89.   A feverish twenty seven month old black female is in excruciating pain. The child has
       hepatomegaly and the spleen is tender. A diagnosis of sickle cell disease is made . The child
       requires immunization to protect her from bacterial septicemia.

90.   A Medical resident must be immunized before she can begin seeing patients at Children's Medical
       Center.

126

A. Pooled gamma globulin   (human)

B. Specific immune globulin
   (human)

C. Transfusion of erythrocytes

D. Bone marrow transplant

E. Fetal thymus transplant

F. Toxoid and specific immune
   globulin (human)

G. Killed virus vaccine and
   specific immune globulin
   (human)

H. Live virus vaccine

I. Purified capsular
   carbohydrate vaccine

J. Thymectomy

K. Specific immune globulin
   (horse)

L. Transfusion of neutrophils

M. Splenectomy

N. Thyroidectomy

O. Killed virus vaccine

P. Platelet infusion

91. A twenty three year old college coed has been exposed to german measles while practice teaching at a local Elementary school. She is newly married.

92. Four year old boy suffers from repeated pyogenic infections. Patient has normal antibody levels and has just successfully recovered from chicken pox.

93. This 37 year old female patient presents with exophthalmus; a diagnosis of hyperthyroidism is made.

94. Forty eight hours after eating home canned green beans, 4 members of the same family develop diplopia. They rapidly progress to respiratory distress due to an ensuing flaccid paralysis.

95. Typhoid Mary, a *Salmonella typhi* chronic carrier, develops aplastic anemia after 3 weeks of chloramphenicol therapy.

96. An eighteen month old child presents with chronic candida infection. The patient has normal phagocytic functions and isoagglutinin levels. Lymph node biopsy reveals acellular paracortical areas.

97. An influenza pandemic is developing in the Far East; the residents of the local nursing home need to be protected.

98. This 14 year old boy was attack by a skunk while camping; Negri bodies were observed in the animal's brain.

99. A veterinary student requires immunization to protest her from Rhabdoviral disease.

100. This twenty-six year old mother of four has acute lymphoblastic leukemia.

KEY

1.	A	21.	B	41.	D	61.	A	81.	I
2.	C	22.	B	42.	B	62.	E	82.	H
3.	C	23.	C	43.	A	63.	E	83.	B
4.	E	24.	C	44.	D	64.	C	84.	A
5.	D	25.	D	45.	D	65.	E	85.	D
6.	B	26.	A	46.	B	66.	D	86.	B
7.	B	27.	C	47.	C	67.	C	87.	E
8.	D	28.	A	48.	C	68.	A	88.	A
9.	E	29.	D	49.	D	69.	E	89.	I
10.	D	30.	B	50.	B	70.	A	90.	H
11.	D	31.	D	51.	D	71.	E	91.	H
12.	C	32.	B	52.	E	72.	E	92.	L
13.	C	33.	C	53.	C	73.	B	93.	J
14.	C	34.	A	54.	A	74.	B	94.	B
15.	C	35.	B	55.	B	75.	E	95.	D
16.	B	36.	D	56.	B	76.	D	96.	E
17.	C	37.	B	57.	D	77.	D	97.	O
18.	D	38.	C	58.	E	78.	A	98.	G
19.	D	39.	D	59.	E	79.	C	99.	O
20.	B	40.	D	60.	E	80.	E	100.	D

REVIEW OF
PATHOGENIC
MICROBIOLOGY

The first portion of this section will deal with infectious diseases by various body systems. This will then be followed by descriptions of the major pathogens encountered in each body region, with particular attention being paid to those of major incidence in the United States of America.

RESPIRATORY TRACT MICROBIOLOGY

The respiratory tract has an enormous normal flora, which extends from the lips to the larynx. The bronchial tree distal to the larynx is usually considered sterile, although microbial agents are continuously impinging upon those surfaces as well. They normally do not colonize, however, and are removed by the mucociliary blanket as it propels upward from the bronchioles. Thus factors that interfere with secretory processes or ciliary action will predispose the host to infections in the lower respiratory tract.

Normal Flora

Most of **the agents are potential pathogens.** Some only express their pathogenicity in immunological compromised hosts; (for example, *Pneumocystis carinii* in AIDS patients); others cause disease when they gain access to areas of the body more susceptible to their deleterious effects. Examples of the latter include *Neisseria meningitidis*, and *Staphylococcus aureus*. The most commonly encountered microorganisms are enumerated below.

Microbial Agents Found in the Upper Respiratory Tract

PROTOZOA	BACTERIA	FUNGI	VIRUSES
Entamoeba	*Streptococcus*	*Candida*	Adeno
Trichomonas	*Staphylococcus*		Herpes
Pneumocystis	*Neisseria*		Rhino
	Corynebacterium		Reo
	Haemophilus		
	Klebsiella		
	Pseudomonas		
	Mycoplasma		

It is perhaps permissible to consider all **normal flora** as agents responsible for **inapparent infections,** as they have colonized the tissues and are multiplying without causing discomfort to their host. In fact in some instances they may be of benefit, as they will limit the growth rate of less desirable inhabitants either through elaboration of products antagonistic to the other microbes or by successful competition for nutrients. Individuals on broad spectrum antibiotic therapy often experience **thrush**, a disease resultant from modification of the flora is caused by *Candida albicans* (*Candida* are resistant to the usually antibiotics).

The **viruses** represent a somewhat different type of inapparent infection in that they grow **within the cells** and may cause some very localized tissue destruction. REO (Respiratory Enteric Orphan) viruses are readily isolated from the upper respiratory tract but have not been convincingly associated with any pathological process. The **adenoviruses** were first isolated from **normal adenoidal tissues**; however, most human serotypes are not associated with disease processes. **Herpesviruses** are sometimes referred to as **latent viruses** in that they persist in the host after an initial infection and recurrent clinical disease may be elicited by various environmental and/or hormonal stimuli.

130

Disease Spectrum

Acute respiratory diseases afflict 200 million people in the United States each year. The clinical pictures that are manifested in the respiratory tract are extremely variable. The diseases may be characterized as to clinical course, pathologic process or anatomic location. As a general rule, **upper** respiratory tract infections are acute processes with short incubation periods and relatively rapid clinical courses; whereas **lower** respiratory diseases of microbial etiology may be either acute (e.g., pneumococcal pneumonia) or chronic, such as mycotic infections or tuberculosis. Chronic diseases are characteized by the development of granulomas, in which the predominate cellular response is mononuclear. Polymorphonuclear leukocytes are the cells that are usually found in acute infectious processes. The most common microbial etiologies of respiratory disease are presented below.

Common Agents of Upper Respiratory Infections

Clinical Illness	Bacteria	Viruses	Fungi
Rhinitis		**Rhinoviruses**[1]	
Stomatitis		**Herpes simplex**	*Candida albicans*
Otitis media and Sinusitis	***Streptococcus pneumoniae*** *Haemophilus influenzae*		
Otitis externa	***Pseudomonas***		*Aspergillus*
Epiglottitis	***Haemophilus influenzae***		
Pharyngitis and Tonsillitis	***Streptococcus pyogenes***	Adenoviruses	*Candida albicans*
Laryngotracheitis (croup)		**Parainfluenza**	
Bronchitis	*Haemophilus influenzae* *Bordetella pertussis in young children*	**Parainfluenza** Respiratory syncytial virus Adenoviruses	

1. The most common agent in each illness category is in **bold face**

Pneumonia

Pneumonia (pneumonitis) is defined as any inflammation of the lung parenchyma diistal to the bronchioles. It may involve the air sacs with exudation into the alveoli or it may be seen as an interstitial lesion, which is the case with most of the viral agents. Bacterial pneumonias are the leading cause of mortality due to infection in the United States, being responsible for over 70,000 deaths per year. Many of the etiologic agents are normal flora of the nasopharynx. *Klebsiella pneumoniae*, for example, is a significant cause of pneumonia in alcoholics although it causes very little clinical disease in individuals with a more intact respiratory apparatus. Many severe diseases result from secondary bacerial invasion following viral infections or whooping cough. The etiology varies with the age of the patient; this is summarized below.

Most Common Causes of Pneumonia

Age	Microorganism
0 - 1 month	Group B streptococci and *E. coli*
1 month - 1 year	Respiratory Syncytial virus (RSV)
1 - 5 years	Parainfluenza virus
5 - 30 years	Mycoplasma (Influenza virus epidemics)
Over 30 years	*Streptococcus pneumoniae*
Debilitated	*Klebsiella pneumoniae*
AIDS at any age	*Pneumocystis carinii*

Viral pneumonias usually take a much more benign course; they are often referred to as "walking pneumonia," meaning the patient is still ambulatory. Differences in bacterial and viral pneumonias are summarized below. *Mycoplasma pneumoniae*, *Coxiella burneti*, and *Chlamydia psittaci* cause a similar mild disease. Many of the differences in symptoms relates to the fact that the viruses and mycoplasma cause an interstitial pneumonitis while most bacterial agents are inhabiting the alveoli and bronchial tree with resultant inflammatory exudation (i.e., sputum) into the airways

Clinical Differentiation of Pneumonias

Characteristic	Bacterial	Viral
Age of Pt.	Adult	Child
Onset	Sudden	Gradual
Fever	High	Moderate
Cough	Productive	Dry
Microbial Site of Replication	Airways	Interstitium
Sputum	Copious; purulent	Moderate; mucoid
Elevated WBC	Common	Rare
Chills	Common	Rare
Pleuritis	Common	Rare
Tachypnea	Common	Rare
Tachycardia	Common	Rare

Complications of Bacterial Pneumonia

The organisms may spread contiguously to involve the pleural space causing pleuritis or empyema (bacteria and WBC in the pleural space). If the organisms become hematogenous they can cause septicemia or may localize in various organs and cause disease there (e.g., meningitis, arthritis, etc.)

Immunity

The major protective immune response is humoral and antibodies act primarily via their opsonic ability. Many of the agents are encapsulated and the IgG and IgM neutralize the anti-phagocytic properties of these carbohydrates. **Pneumovax** is a mixture of capsular carbohydrates from 23 serotypes of *S. pneumoniae*. It is presently recommended for patients particularly susceptible to pneumococcal disease because of age, underlying disease (e.g. sickle cell disease) or immune deficiency.

Diagnosis of Bacterial Pneumonia

A Gram stain can be valuable as an early guide to therapy. Also the age of the patient should be taken into consideration. Sputum samples should be plated on blood-containing media (blood agar or chocolate agar). A good sputum specimen will contain PMNs and a relatively pure microbial population; samples from the upper respiratory tract (saliva) will have numerous squamous epithelial cells and a variety of microbes present. Antibiotic sensitivity should be done on the microorganism isolated from the sample.

Therapy for Pneumonias

The patient should be treated with aspirin to help with the fever and discomfort; oxygen and external cooling may also be required. The following are drugs of choice for the agents listed (these same antibiotics could be used for treatment of infections caused by the same organisms in other parts of the body).

Streptococcus	Penicillin
Staphylococcus	Penicillinase-resistant beta lactam antibiotic (EG., Oxacillin, Methicillin; methicillin- resistant *S. aureus* (MRSA) can be treated with Vancomycin
Mycoplasma	Erythromycin
Legionella	Erythromycin
Chlamydia	Erythromycin or tetracycline
Escherichia	3rd generation cephalosporin
Klebsiella	3rd generation cephalosporin plus an aminoglycoside
Respiratory syncytial virus	Ribavirin via aerosol
Influenza virus	Amantadine
Pneumocystis	Trimethoprim plus sulfamethoxazole

SEPSIS

The terms bacteremia and septicemia are sometimes used interchangeably. Transient bacteremias occur every day. When it becomes clinically noticeable then it is usually called a septicemia. Septicemia is the 13th leading cause of death in the United States.

Predisposing Factors

Primary conditions that can lead to septicemia include urinary tract infection, burns, prolonged intravenous therapy and septic abortion. Underlying diseases that predispose to septicemia and shock include AIDS, leukemia, diabetes, cirrhosis, and sickle cell anemia.

Symptoms

Fever may be the only clinical manifestation of septicemia; it is usually associated with chills, malaise, sweating, headache, abdominal pain, myalgia and arthralgia.

Splenomegaly is a common presentation. There is a particular syndrome that is associated with **meningococcemia,** i.e. the **Waterhouse-Friderichsen syndrome** (adrenalcortical necrosis). These patients also usually have a petechial rash. Many infectious agents can cause disseminated intravascular coagulopathy (DIC) and septic shock with associated hypotension.

Hematogenous dissemination can result in secondary foci of infection in the CNS, cardiovascular, and renal tissues; arthritis may also occur.

Etiologies of Septicemia

Group B streptococci and **E. coli** predominate in the neonatal period. **Pneumococcus** and **Neisseria meningitidis** are among the most common in children. **Staphylococci** and enteric bacteria occur in patients who acquire bacteremia in hospitals.

The most common cause of septicemia in asplenic or sickle cell patients is **Streptococcus pneumoniae.** **Staphylococci** are the main cause of septicemia following a surgical procedure.

Escherichia coli is the most common cause of gram negative bacteremia/septicemia; the origin of the microbe is the GI or GU tract. The signs/symptoms include shaking and chills, prostration and hypotension (LPS shock). Gram negative organisms can also be introduced by needle. This is an etiology that might be expected in an IV drug user. The most common agent here is also *Escherichia coli.* Other etiological agents of Gram negative bacteremia include *Klebsiella, Pseudomonas,* and *Proteus.* The most comon cause of Gram negative septicemia in a burn patient is **Pseudomonas.** If the patient is an army recruit the organism would be **Neisseria meningitidis.** Complications of bacteremia and septic shock include; meningitis, disseminated infection, and endotoxin shock.

Diagnosis of Bacteremia/Sepsis

Fever and **hypotension** are the biggest clues for diagnosing bacteremia. The recommendation is to do repeated blood cultures throughout a 24 hour period at 4 hour intervals. Serial blood cultures of 10-15 ml should be drawn during febrile periods.

Therapy of Bacteremia/Sepsis

Since this is a rapidly evolving condition, aggressive intervention is needed to avoid having the patient die. Gram stain of purulent exudate may help determine the portal of entry and what the agent might be. Antibiotic susceptibility testing should be done. Use the intravenous route and continue therapy two weeks.

Endocarditis/Myocarditis

Staphylococcus aureus is the most common cause of **acute bacterial endocarditis** in normal heart tissue. The organisms that causes **subacute bacterial endocarditis** (SBE) are *viridans streptococci.* These organisms attack previously damaged heart tissue. This usually infects secondarily to a previous infection. Some of the predisposing factors are Rheumatic Heart Disease, valvular damage or prosthetic valves. Laboratory diagnosis of SBE depends on demonstration of alpha hemolytic streptococci that are not inhibited by **optochin.**

Coxsackie group **B** viruses are the most common viral cause of **myocarditis.** They also cause pleurodynia characterized by fever and severe pleuritic chest pain. Group A Coxsackie viruses are primarily associated with herpangina which is characterized by fever, sore throat, and tender vesicles in the oropharynx.

Septic Arthritis/Osteomyelitis

The same agents that predominate in neonatal pneumonias and meningitides are also seen in these consequences of septicemia, i.e. **group B streptococci and** *E. coli.* In older infants and children to the age of five *Haemophilus influenzae* **type** b is found most frequently as a cause of septic arthritis; this will likely decline as the vaccine becomes more widely used. *Staphylococcus aureus* is the most common cause of **septic arthritis and osteomyelitis** in all other age groups with perhaps the exception of *Neisseria gonorrhoeae* arthritis as a serious sequela of gonococcal infections in sexually active individuals.

135

PURULENT MENINGITIDES

The presence of large amounts of pus characterize most of the bacterial meningitides, in distinction to those of fungal or viral etiology where the inflammatory response is primarily lymphocytic or granulomatous. Purulent meningitis presents a real medical emergency due to the fulminate nature of the disease which develops. The infection may be limited to the leptomeninges or the brain parenchyma may also be infected (meningoencephalitis). The viral diseases are called **aseptic** because the etiological agent is not recovered from the patient by standard bacteriological techniques, not because the agent is not present in the lesion.

ETIOLOGY

Bacterial meningitis most commonly results from **hematogenous dissemination** of an organism which is either a member of the normal flora or is causing an infection in another part of the body, usually the lungs. The age of the host and his immunologic status have a major bearing on the type of organism causing the disease. Bacterial meningitis in neonates is usually caused by *E. coli* or group B streptococci. Both are normal inhabitants of the birth canal and may colonize the skin or gastrointestinal tract of the infant.

The **oropharynx** is usually the source of organisms causing bacterial meningitis in children greater than 2 months of age and in adults. The most common etiological agents of acute bacterial meningitis as they are distributed in different age groups is presented below. Fatality rates vary with the agent and the age of the patient but in general are highest in neonates (over 50%) and the elderly. A 10 to 20 percent mortality is seen in the other age groups.

Common Causes of Purulent Meningitis

Age	Microbial Etiology	Approximate Incidence[1]
Less than 2 months	Group B streptococci	40
	E. coli	30
2 to 60 months	*H. influenzae*	60[2]
5 to 40	*N. meningitidis*	45
over 40	*S. pneumoniae*	50

[1]These figures are the number of cases caused by that agent per 100 in that age group.
[2]The introduction of the HIB conjugate vaccine is causing this number to decrease. In the next few years the meningococcus or the pneumococcus will likely take over.

Brain abscesses may develop from hematogenous dissemination of organisms but more often are the result of trauma (during birth, accident, or surgery) or by direct extension from contiguous tissue such as the sinuses and mastoids. The causative organisms include peptostreptococci, staphylococci, *Bacteroides spp,* and Group A or D streptococci. ***Staphylococcus aureus*** and ***S epidermidis*** are the leading causes of brain abscesses following trauma (accidental or surgical).

MANIFESTATIONS OF DISEASE

The most common findings in purulent meningitis are **fever** (often over 105° F, particularly in infants) **headache** and **nuchal rigidity** caused by paraspinal muscle spasms resulting from meningeal irritation. The increased intracranial pressure which develops as a result of the acute inflammatory response may cause bulging of the fontanelle. A list of the major symptoms of meningitis are presented in the Table below. The clinical course is highly variable being dependent upon the agent, and the age and associated immunologic status of the host. However, the disease is usually acute and death can occur within a few hours of the onset of symptoms.

Clinical Findings Suggestive of Meningitis

Symptom	Comment
Fever	100 - 106°F
Headache	Generalized, persistent and extremely painful
Stiff Neck	Positive Brudzinski [1] and Kernig [2] signs [3]
Decreased mental function	Lethargy, confusion, delirium, coma
Vomiting, anorexia	Seen in neonates

(1) Resistance to neck flexion when in a supine position with knees raised

(2) Inability to straighten the leg when supine and thigh is perpendicular to body

(3) These will be absent in neonates

Post-meningitis sequelae are uncommon except in the neonatal patient, where approximately 50 percent will exhibit either motor or intellectual impairment. It is important to follow these patients for a few years after their acute disease in order that appropriate rehabilitative action can be taken should any dysfunction surface.

DIAGNOSIS

Cerebrospinal Fluid (CSF)

In patients with brain abscesses this examination reveals little and may in fact be contraindicated due to the potential for mechanical injury to the brain as a result of its displacement caused by intracranial and spinal column pressure differentials. In patients with purulent meningitis where a spinal tap is indicated the following abnormalities will be found.

1. The presence of **neutrophils** - 400 to 20,000cmm, the observation of large numbers of lymphocytes would suggest mycobacterial, mycotic or viral meningitis.
2. **Glucose concentrations significantly lower** than that in blood. The glucose is utilized by the phagocytic cellsas well as by most of the bacterial organisms causing meningitis Viral disease does not cause a decrease in glucose.
3. **Elevated protein concentration** - associated with the inflammatory response.
4. **The presence of bacteria** detected by Gram stain.
5. **The presence of bacterial products** - most of the pathogens are encapsulated and the development of sensitive tests (e.g. ELISA) has permitted the identification of capsular antigens in spinal fluid.

Bacterial cultures

In all cases it is imperative that CSF cultures be performed, and antibiotic sensitivities be determined on the organism isolated. It is common to centrifuge the specimen before inoculating the media. Blood cultures should also be done.

THERAPY

The fulminating nature of bacterial meningitis precludes any delay in the institution of antimicrobic therapy. The age of the patient is a major guideline in the selection of the appropriate antimicrobial. Ampicillin should be given to the very young (in the case of *H. influenzae* some pediatricians add chloramphenicol to cover the 15-20% of strains that contain a b lactamase encoding plasmid) Penicillin is the drug to give to patients above 5 years of age. Modifications in antibiotic therapy should be considered after culture and sensitivity testing is completed.

The intravenous route of drug administration should be used as the patient's condition often compromises absorption from the gut or intramuscular depot. Large "loading" doses are necessary as very few antibiotics cross the blood-brain barrier readily (an exception is chloramphenicol) and it is imperative to achieve bactericidal concentrations in the CSF rapidly. Treatment should be continued for at least 1 week after symptoms have subsided and for longer periods in neonates.

ENTERIC DISEASES

Acute gastrointestinal infection ranks as one of the most prevalent of ills which affects mankind, and in its complex interactions with malnutrition, this group of disorders ranks high among the killing diseases of childhood being responsible for 3-5 million deaths per year world wide.

NORMAL FLORA OF THE GASTROINTESTINAL TRACT

Composition. The feces of normal adults contain from 10^{11} to 10^{12} viable bacteria/gram. The majority of these bacteria are found in the colon. The fluid contents of the small intestine contain between 10^2 to 10^3 bacteria/ml, and in the terminal ileum the count usually does not exceed 10^7. The bacterial flora of the gastrointestinal tract is established within several weeks after birth and remains relatively stable for life. The dominant bacteria in feces are non-sporeforming anaerobic bacilli (*Bacteroides*) although coliforms, such as *Escherichia coli* and other members of the family *Enterobacteriaceae* are also normally present.

Transient organisms are seen in the stomach and upper small intestine, whereas, organisms which adhere to and colonize the mucosal surface are observed in the distal ileum and large bowel. Obligate anaerobes outnumber facultative organisms at least 1000:1. The indigenous flora of the large bowel is diverse in compostion although it is predominated by Gram-negative organisms; e.g., *Bacteroides, Fusobacterium* and coliforms. Gram-positive cocci and bacilli are also present, including lactobacilli, *Peptostreptococcus*, enterococci, and clostridia.

Microorganisms Normally Found in The Gastrointestinal Tract

Stomach and Upper Small Bowel (These transients are found throughout the GI tract)

Lactobacilli
Streptococci
Bifidobacteria
Clostridia
Veillonella
Coliforms
Yeasts

Distal ileum

Bacteroides

Large Bowel and feces

Peptostreptococcus
Peptococcus
Propionibacterium
Bacteroides
Fusobacterium

In addition to bacteria, certain parasites and viruses are classified as enteric agents. Although many of the respiratory viruses may produce gastrointestinal symptoms, two major groups associated with viral gastroenteritis are the Rotaviruses and the Norwalk agent. The parasites *Entamoeba histolytica* and *Giardia lamblia* are primary pathogens of the gastrointestinal tract. Other parasites, including *Trichinella spiralis*, *Balantidium coli*, *Schistosoma* and *Strongyloides stercoralis* may induce enteric disease during certain phases of their infective cycle in man.

Function

Normal flora may enhance the host defense mechanisms by 1) production of bacteriocins and antibiotics active against potential pathogens; 2) competition for nutrients; 3) occupation of the intestinal mucosal surface, thereby preventing exogenous pathogens from attaching and 4) serving as a constant source of immunogens, continually priming the local and systemic immune systems. Two negative aspects of the gastrointestinal flora are 1) a source of antigens which induce endotoxin tolerance and 2) large numbers of organisms potentially dangerous when bowel perforation occurs or the host become severely immunologically compromised.

An important factor in establishing enteric infection is the ability of the parasite to adhere to host mucosal surfaces. The adherence of bacteria to animal cells is dependent on specific recognition systems Receptors on the membranes of tissue cells interact with specific ligands on surfaces of bacteria. Lipoteichoic acid (LTA), fimbrial protein, colonizing factor antigen, and other microbial surface proteins are thought to serve as ligands involved in host cell adhesion. Animal strains of *E. coli* possessing K88 and K89 antigens may bind to host cells via galactose or N-acetylgalactosamine moieties, respectively. Human strains of *E. coli* seem to possess a mannose-specific lectin-like substance that binds the organisms via fimbriae to mannose residues on epithelial cells.

Toxins of Enteric Bacilli

Endotoxin, the LPS moiety of the Gram-negative cell wall, is highly toxic. The biological effects of bacterial endotoxins are myriad (see Table below), although no clearcut molecular-biological basis for their activities is known. Many effects of endotoxin appear to be mediated through host humoral and cellular responses. The morbidity and mortality associated with many infections caused by Gram-negative bacteria are considered related to the endotoxins present in the cell walls of these bacteria.

Biological Effects Induced by Bacterial Endotoxins

Pyrogenicity
Lethal shock
Adjuvancy
Shwartzman phenomenon
Tumor necrosis
Leukopenia - leukocytosis
Hypotension
Plasminogen activation
Enhancement of nonspecific resistance

Mitogenic for B lymphocytes
Increases interferon production
Release of colony-stimulating factor
Complement activation
Hageman factor activation
Stimulation of prostaglandin synthesis

Enterotoxins are usually protein substances that exert their toxic effect specifically in the small intestine. The **choleragen of *V. cholerae*** is the prototype of bacterial enterotoxins. A number of enterics have been shown to produce enterotoxic materials which cause large amounts of fluid and electrolytes to be secreted into the intestinal lumen, without demonstrable gastrointestinal histopathology .

140

Spectrum of Enteric Diseases

Diseases that affect the gastrointestinal tract of man are diverse and multifaceted. In a few cases, the pathogenesis is well understood, although most of the syndromes have only recently been studied in experimental animal models. The spectrum of microbial enteric infections is presented below.

TYPE OF INTESTINAL BACTERIAL INFECTIONS

Type of Infection	Microorganisms	Virulence Factors	Clinical Features		
				Stools	
			Fever	water	pus
Bacteria attach to epithelium of small intestine and cause **watery diarrhea** by forming an enterotoxin which induces fluid loss from epithelial cells	*Vibrio cholerae* *E. coli*	Adhesin Enterotoxin ADP ribosylates an adenylate cyclase regulatory protein, causing an increase in enzyme activity	No No		Yes
Microorganism attaches to and penetrates epithelial cells of large intestine or ileum causing **bloody diarrhea** by killing cells	*E. coli* *Campylobacter jejuni* *Yersinia enterocolitica* *Shigella spp.** *Salmonella spp.**	Adhesin Hemin binding protein in outer membrane coats cells which are then taken up to enterocytes Cytotoxin kills enterocytes	Yes Yes		No
Bacteria attach to and penetrate epithelium of small intestine. Invade subepithelial tissues, cause ulceration and spread systemically	*Salmonella typhi* *Salmonella cholerasuis*	Adhesin Vi surface antigen Microbes survives in phagocytes by inhibiting oxidative metabolism and production of toxic oxygen metabolites Endotoxin	Yes No		No

* Only these 2 affect large intestine; the rest are pathogens of the small intestine.

141

Laboratory Diagnosis

Laboratory diagnostic procedures include microscopic examination, culture, toxin detection, and serologic procedures. The relative value of each is different for the various etiologies.

Treatment

In most gastrointestinal infections the goal of treatment is relief of symptoms, with particular attention to maintaining fluid and electrolyte balance. The effect of common antidiarrheal medications such as bismuth compounds (Pepto Bismol) or antispasmotics (lomotil) is variable depending on the etiology. In general, they may be helpful for the watery diarrhea caused by enterotoxins, but not for dysentery caused by mucosal invasion, and antispasmotics may be harmful in the latter instance. Antimicrobial agents are usually not indicated for self-limited watery diarrhea, but are required for more severe dysenteric infections. Some enteric infections, such as typhoid fever, are always treated with antimicrobics.

Antibiotic-induced Gastrointestinal Disease

The prolonged administration of antibiotics, particularly those with an extended spectrum, may alter the existing balance in the normal flora and give minor members of that population (that are resistant to the antibiotic) an opportunity to increase in numbers to such an extent that they will produce disease. Two diseases deserve mention.

Thrush, a *Candida albicans* infection of the oral cavity, can occur following the use of broad spectrum antibiotics, particularly via the per os route. This same yeast infection occurs in the very young and in immuno-compromised patients of any age. Parenteral antibiotic administration may permit the overgrowth of candida cells in the vaginal tract or in the anal area, with resultant irritation and disease (e.g., candidal vaginitis).

Pseudomembranous colitis results from an overproliferation of the obligate anaerobic organism *Clostridium difficile.* This organism may be resistant to several antibiotics that act on other members of the colonic flora, thus giving it a selective advantage. In the presence of antibiotic therapy with, for example, **clindamycin**, the clostridia reproduce and elaborate a potent enterotoxin that produces diarrhea with WBC infiltration and hemorrhagic necrosis of the intestinal mucosa. **Vancomycin** is the drug of choice, although merely withholding the offending antibiotic often is successful.

Food Poisoning

Many gastrointestinal infections involve food as a vehicle of transmission. The term "food poisoning" however, is usually reserved for instances in which a single meal can be incriminated as the source. This usually arises when multiple cases of the disease develop among persons whose only common experience is a shared meal.

The most common causes of food poisoning are shown in table below. Some are not infections but intoxications caused by ingestion of a toxin produced by bacteria in the food before it was eaten. Intoxications generally have shorter incubation periods than infections and may involve extra-intestinal symptoms (for example, the neurologic damage in botulism). Infectious food poisoning does not differ from endemic diarrheal infections caused by the same species. The length of the incubation period and the severity of the symptoms are generally related to the number of organisms in the infecting dose.

CLINICAL AND EPIDEMIOLOGIC FEATURES OF FOOD POISONING

Etiology	Incubation Period (hr)	Clinical Findings	Characteristic Foods
Intoxications			
Bacillus cereus	1-6	Vomiting, diarrhea	Rice
Staphylococcus aureus	1-6	Vomiting	Meats, custards, salads
Clostridium botulinum	12-72	Neuromuscular paralysis	Improperly preserved vegetables, meats
Infections			
Cl. perfringens	12-24	Watery diarrhea	Meat, poultry
Salmonella spp.	6-48	Gastroenteritis	Poultry products
Shigella spp.	12-48	Dysentery	Variable
Vibrio parahemolyticus	12-24	Watery diarrhea	Shellfish
Trichinella spiralis	3-30 days	Fever, myalgia	Pork
Hepatitis A	10-50 days	Hepatitis	Shellfish

SEXUALLY TRANSMITTED DISEASES

The incidence of sexually transmitted diseases (STD) has increased alarmingly in the last 2 decades, and has now reached epidemic proportions. The incidence of the major venereal diseases is presented in the table below. The most serious complications of these diseases include infertility, congenital abnormalities, ectopic pregnancy and abortion.

The Major Pathogens and Their Estimated Frequencies in the United States

Disease	Pathogen	Annual cases
Condylomata acuminata (Genital warts)	Papillomavirus	10,000,000
Non-gonococcal urethritis	*Chlamydia trachomatis*	4,000,000
Gonorrhea	*Neisseria gonorrhoeae*	2,000,000
Genital herpes	Herpesvirus type II	500,000
Syphilis	*Treponema pallidum*	150,000
Cervical carcinoma	Papillomavirus	20,000

Epidemiology and Etiology

These diseases are contracted during sexual intercourse. The increase in oral and/or anal sexual contact has changed the method of spread as well as the types of diseases transmitted. Several enteric diseases are now considered STDs among homosexual males. It is not uncommon for a patient to have more than one STD at the same time. A partial list grouped by sexual incidence is tabulated below.

Sexually Transmitted Pathogens of Women

Microbe	Disease
Gardnerella vaginalis	Vaginitis
Group B streptococci	Neonatal sepsis and meningitis
Trichomonas	Vaginitis
Candida albicans	Vulvovaginitis

Sexually Transmitted Among Homosexual Men

Shigella spp.	Shigellosis
Campylobacter fetus	Enteritis and proctitis
Herpesvirus hominis, type II	Genital herpes
Hepatitis B	Hepatitis
Entamoeba histolytica	Amebiasis
Giardia lamblia	Giardiasis

Prevention and Control

The condom is the most effective means of **protection** against venereal disease. Unfortunately, individuals who need protection the most (those with multiple sex partners) are the least likely to use them.

Control of STD is best accomplished by diagnosis and treatment of patients and their sexual contacts. Prompt reporting of all cases to the appropriate health agency is imperative if a thorough epidemiological survey and partner contact is to be achieved. At least 3 factors are operating to confound attempts at the control of these diseases. First, many patients are reluctant to seek medical assistance due to embarrassment, guilt, fear of complications in their personal lives, etc. Secondly, many cases are asymptomatic, particularly in females. Finally, **treatment must be sufficient to cure** the disease. Whenever possible a single dose therapy should be employed as the patient's continued self-treatment will probably stop when the symptoms moderate, which very likely will not coincide with a bacteriological cure.

Common Presenting Complaints

Urethral Discharge of purulent material is seen in infections with the **gonococcus, *C. trachomatis, C. albicans, T. vaginalis*** and type II herpes virus. A burning pain is usually associated with urination.

A copious vaginal discharge, characterized by the presence of large numbers of neutrophils and an offensive odor, is seen in women infected with many of the same agents that cause urethritis in males. **Gardnerella vaginalis** also causes a vaginitis; characteristics of the latter include by a fishy odor and the presence of "clue" cells (i.e., sloughed epithelial cells with adherent gram negative rods).

Skin lesions may be of 2 types, either as a rash or an ulcer. **Rashes** are seen in candidiasis and in secondary syphilis. **Ulcerative** lesions occur in syphilis, and genital herpes.

Complications

The serious consequences of STDs are manifold. They may result from;
1) **contiguous** spread of the infection to involve the reproductive organs,
2) **hematogenous** dissemination of the microorganism to other organ systems,
3) **infection of the infant** either during pregnancy or while passing through the birth canal. A list of the more common complications is presented in the table below. **Salpingitis** (inflammation of the fallopian tubes) is probably the most serious manifestation of STD in females. It can lead to infertility (nearly 20% in women with 1 or more cases of salpingitis) and ectopic pregnancies with resultant fetal death and potential maternal mortality.

Infant morbidity and mortality due to ***T. pallidum*** and the gonococci is quite low in the United States due to the fact that pregnant women are routinely tested and treated for these agents; however, congenital and perinatal diseases caused by **cytomegalovirus, herpes virus**, *C. trachomatis* and **Group B streptococci** are of considerable importance.

At least 2 malignancies are thought to be associated with STDs of viral etiology. Cervical carcinoma has been suggested as a sequela of **Papilloma virus** infections. Hepatocellular carcinoma has been linked to **hepatitis type B viral disease**. Acquired Immune Deficiency Syndrome (AIDS) is another human affliction which occurs as a sequela of a sexually transmitted infection caused by the human immunodeficiency virus..

Complications of Sexually Transmitted Diseases

Method of Dissemination	Disease
Contiguous	Salpingitis Epididymitis
Hematogenous	Hepatitis Meningitis Arthritis
Congenital	Abortion, birth defects, etc.
Perinatal infections	Conjunctivitis Pneumonia Sepsis Meningitis

Miscellaneous Genitourinary Pathogens

Escherichia coli is the most common cause of uncomplicated urinary tract infections (cystitis and pyelonephritis), causing over 80 %of all disease. Klebsiella pneumoniae is #2 at 5-10%. The same two agents predominate in prostatitis. **Adenovirus type 2** causes an **acute hemnorhagic cystitis in young children.** Patients with urinary tract abnormalities that interfere with urine flow are likely to experience chronic and/or recurrent infections. Hospitalized patients are susceptible to nosocomial infections with agents other than E. coli, although this agent still predominates in most urinary catheter-induced cases.

PRINCIPAL MICROORGANISMS INFECTING THE HUMAN FETUS

	Microorganisms	Effect
VIRUSES	Rubella virus	Abortion Still birth Malformations
	Cytomegalovirus	Malformations
	Human Immuno- deficiency Virus	AIDS
BACTERIA	Treponema pallidum	Stillbirth, malformation
	Listeria monocytogenes	Meningoencephalitis
PROTOZOA	Toxoplasma gondii	Stillbirth, CNS disease

The mnemonic for these agents is TORCHES

    TOxoplasma
    Rubella
    Cytomegalovirus
    Human Immunodeficiency virus
    Herpes
    Syphilis

THE GRAM STAIN

The Gram stain aids in the identification of bacteria according to their size, shape and grouping by rendering them more visible. It also helps identify them by dividing the eubacteria into Gram positive or negative organisms. The cell wall composition of Gram negative bacteria differs from that of Gram positive. Since Gram negative bacteria have a high lipid content of their cell walls, one theory holds that the decolorizer (acetone or ethanol) solubilizes the cell wall thus reaching the crystal violet. In the cell wall of Gram positive organisms, the decolorizer is unable to act as a solvent thus the crystal violet remains.

Step	Reagent
1.	Crystal violet (c.v.)
2.	Sodium bicarbonate
3.	Gram's iodine
4.	Acetone
5.	Safranin

Appearance of organisms, step by step:

Gram Positive	Gram Negative
1. purple	purple
2. purple;alkalinized	purple;alkalinized
3. purple;fixes c.v. in cell	purple;fixes c.v. in cell
4. purple	colorless; c.v. washes out because cell wall (lipid) soluble in acetone -thus the organisms are unstained again
5. purple	red/pink

Mycoplasma do not have a cell wall. Their gram reaction would be

_____.

Age can cause conversion from Gram positive to negative. What technical errors in the staining procedure could do the same?

1. _____

2. _____

3. _____

The thick spore coat is resistant to the penetration of dyes. They will appear blue/red/colorless in a Gram stain?

MORPHOLOGY AND GRAM REACTION OF SOME BACTERIA OF MEDICAL IMPORTANCE

Gram +   Gram −

COCCI

Staphylococcus   Neisseria
Streptococcus   Veillonella(2)

BACILLI

Bacillus(1)   Escherichia
Clostridium(1,2) Klebsiella
Corynebacterium   Proteus
Listeria   Pseudomonas
Mycobacterium   Salmonella
                  Shigella
                  Brucella
                  Francisella
                  Yersinia
                  Haemophilus
                  Bordetella
                  Bacteroides(2)

SPIROCHETES

Borrelia(2)
Leptospira
Treponema(2)

1. only sporeforming pathogens
2. only obligate anaerobic pathogens in list

Generalities That Can Be Draw From Gram Reaction Table

Generality	Exceptions
All cocci are Gram positive	Neisseria, Veillonella
All rods are Gram negative	Bacillus, Clostridia, Corynebacteria, Listeria, Mycobacteria
All pathogens are facultative anaerobes	Clostridia, Bacteroides (obligate anaerobes)
Only bacilli have flagella	None

PROPERTIES OF
A- B TOXINS

Toxin	Structure*	Enzymatic		Biologic Effects
		Activity	Substrate	
Diphtheria toxin	A–B	NADase	Elongation factor II	⬇ Stop protein synthesis (ADP-ribosylate EF-2)
Pseudomonas exotoxin A	↓		↓	
Cholera toxin	A–B$_5$		Adenylate cyclase-regulatory protein	⬆ Increases adenylate cyclase activity
E. coli Heat-labile enterotoxin				
Pertussis toxin	↓	↓	↓	
Botulinum toxin	A–B	Not known	Not known	⬇ Depresses presynaptic acetylcholine release from peripheral neurons
Tetanus toxin	↓			⬇ Depresses neurotransmitter (glycine) release from inhibitory neurons
Shigella toxin	A–B$_5$	↓	↓	⬇ Inhibits protein synthesis

* A is active (toxic) moiety, B is binding protein

PROPERTIES OF
SPECIFIC PATHOGENS

GRAM POSITIVE COCCI

STREPTOCOCCUS GENUS

I. General Characteristics

A. Some have capsules (Group A = hyaluronic acid)
B. Production of hemolysis
   1. _-hemolytic (viridans)
   2. _-hemolytic (complete)
   3. q-hemolytic (none)
C. Catalase negative
D. Penicillin = Drug of Choice

The drug of choice for most streptococcal

infections is _____.

STREPTOCOCCUS PNEUMONIAE

I. General Characteristics

A. bile, optochin, detergents lyse colonies
B. alpha hemolytic; optochin sensitive
C. Drug of choice = penicillin

Artificial, actively acquired immunity

against pneumococcal pneumonia is readily

induced by a vaccine composed of

II. Antigenic Structure

A. Capsular polysaccharide = 75-80 serological types
   1. SSS - specific soluble substance = quellung rx (capsule swelling)
   2. protective antibody = opsonin
   3. Vaccine is composed of SSS from the most prevalent 23 types

_____.

III. Distribution

A. Normal flora; common cause of lobar pneumonia in alcoholics, and as secondary invader following viral infections (e.g., influenza) Hematogenous spread may result in meningitis in debilitated adults.

The pneumococcus is alpha/beta/gamma

hemolytic.

IV. Bacterial Factors Involved in Pathogenicity

A. Prime virulence factor = Capsule - antiphagocytic - content of vaccine (Pneumovac) - confers opsonic immunity

151

BETA-HEMOLYTIC STREPTOCOCCI

I. Antigens used for Identification
(bacterial cell wall antigens)

A. Group-specific C Antigens
   1. carbohydrate
   2. divide organisms into groups A-O;
      A is sensitive to bacitracin

B. Type-specific M Antigens (protein)
   1. subdivide group A into 50 + types
   2. antiphagocytic - virulence factor
   3. immunity is type specific

II. Other Surface Components

A. Hyaluronic acid capsule = antiphagocytic CHO; not antigenic
B. Lipoteichoic acid = important in
   adherence to epithelial cells

III. Extracellular Products

A. Erythrogenic toxin (pyrogenic exotoxin) - produced by lysogenic
   strains of group A
   1. erythema and edema
   2. three immunological types (A-C)
   3. positive Dick test indicates sus-
      ceptibility to Scarlet fever

B. Streptolysin O (oxygen labile; sulf
   hydryl activated)
   1. antigenic - used to detect anti-
      body resulting from infection (ASO)
   2. leukotoxic - cytolytic

C. Streptolysin S (oxygen stable; serum
   required for synthesis)
   1. responsible of hemolysis of
      surface colonies on blood agar
   2. non-antigenic
   3. leukotoxic

D. DNAse
   1. 4 immunologic types (A,B,C,D) -
      type B used to measure antibody
      resulting from infection

E. Streptokinase (Fibrinolysin) -
   converts plasminogen to plasmin

F. Hyaluronidase (spreading factor)

Antigens of importance in the serologic

identification of beta hemolytic

streptococci include

A. group specific C carbohydrate

B. type specific M protein

C. both

D. neither

(answer at bottom of page)

Antiphagocytic surface components

of group A streptococci include

A. hyaluronic acid

B. M protein

C. both

D. neither

(answer at bottom of page)

> Streptococcal pili contain two
> important virulence factors:
> lipoteichoic acid = adherence
> M protein = anti-phagocytic.

(answers to both = C)

152

IV. Types of Diseases

A. Group A (S. pyogenes) acute infections
1. streptococcal pharyngitis (with toxemia = scarlet fever)
2. pneumonia
3. puerperal sepsis
4. erysipelas, impetigo

B. Group A post-infection sequelae
1. acute glomerulonephritis - associated with skin or upper respiratory tract infections
   a) one + weeks after infection
   b) nephritogenic strains (e.g., types 4, 12, 49)
   c) may be antigen-antibody reaction resulting in binding of complement ("lumpy-bumpy" deposition of Ig in basement membrane)
2. acute rheumatic fever - associated with upper respiratory tract infection only: strep M protein cross reacts with heart tissue

C. Non-group A Diseases
1. Caries - plaque caused by adherent dextrans of S. mutans; glucan formed from sucrose by glucosyl transferase; may also predispose to peridontal disease
2. Subacute endocarditis (oral and enteric strep); alpha hemolytic
3. Meningitis and septicemia (enteric strep such as S. agalactiae = group B) in neonates

PEPTOCOCCI, PEPTOSTREPTOCOCCI

I. Obligate anaerobes

II. Mixed infections

III. Pulmonary abscesses by aspiration from oral cavity

(answer is E)

Non-suppurative sequalae of group A streptococcal infections include

A. Scarlet fever

B. erysipelas

C. puerperal fever

D. caries

E. Rheumatic fever

(answer at bottom of page, left side)

```
Rheumatic Fever Symptoms
  Pericarditis
  Arthritis
  Chorea
  SubQ nodules
  Elevated ASO
```

Two streptococcal organisms are commonly associated with meningitis. Complete the table below.

	Patient group	Streptococcal species
example -	kids with caries	S. mutans
	neonates	
	elder	

153

STAPHYLOCOCCUS AUREUS

I. General Characteristics
A. beta hemolytic, facultative aerobe
B. golden pigment
C. coagulase produced
D. catalase positive

II. Surface Antigens
A. capsular antigen - antiphagocytic,
B. protein A-antiphagocytic, reacts with Fc portion of Ig

III. Extracellular substances
A. coagulase
B. alpha toxin - hemolytic, leukotoxic
C. enterotoxin - exotoxin
   1. resistant to boiling
   2. resistant to proteolytic enzymes
   3. incubation period 2-4 hrs for symptoms of food poisoning
   4. toxin ingested preformed
   5. causes nausea, vomiting, diarrhea
D. penicillinase
E. pyrogenic exotoxins (toxic shock)
F. exfoliatin

IV. Types of Infections
A. Most common - pimples, boils, carbuncles, furuncles
B. Most dangerous - septicemia, endocarditis, meningitis, pneumonia, abscesses, osteomyelitis
C. Other diseases - food poisoning (2-4 hr incubation), nosocomial infections post-surgery, scalded skin syndrome in neonates (exotoxin = exfoliatin), Toxic Shock Syndrome (Pyrogenic toxins A-C)

V. Diagnosis
A. Organism isolated on selective media such as Mannitol Salt Agar
B. Demonstrate beta hemolysis
C. Test for production of coagulase and/or DNAse
D. If concerned with hospital epidemic, do bacteriophage typing

VI. Therapy
Because of high incidence of beta lactamase producers (plasmid encoded) start with oxacillin, cefotaxime, or another enzyme-resistant drug

Major Causes of Skin Infections

Staphylococcus aureus	Bullous impetigo Folliculitis(1) Furuncles Carbuncles
Streptococcus pyogenes	Erysipelas Cellulitis Pyoderma (Streptococcal impetigo)

(1) *Propionibacterium* is associated with acne but the primary etiology is unknown.

Staphylococcal **protein A** acts as an **anti-opsonin** by reacting with antibody molecules at the Fab/Fc portion.

> Staphylococci can colonize normal heart valves; alpha streptococci only grow on damaged or prosthetic ones.

An Intoxicating Story

Staphylococcal food poisoning is due to ingestion of preformed enterotoxin, thus the disease has a short/long incubation period.

Foods commonly incriminated include

1. cooked meats like ham = 40%
2. potato salad = 20%
3. baked foods = 10%
4. poultry = 10%

154

GRAM NEGATIVE COCCI

NEISSERIA

I. General Characteristics of Genus

A. Most species are normal human flora (NOT gonococcus)
B. Pathogens occur in vivo inside PMNs
C. Pathogens (fastidious) - grow on chocolate or Thayer-Martin agar, 37C, 10% CO_2, produce indophenol oxidase which is useful in identification of colonies. Produce IgA1 protease.
D. Killed rapidly by drying, sunlight, UV, moist heat at 55 C, phenol
E. Penicillin sensitive: a few strains have plasmid directed beta lactamase

The drug of choice for neisserial

infections is _____.

NEISSERIA MENINGITIDIS

I. Antigenic Structure
A. There are 4 serogroup-specific capsular polysaccharides (A-D)
   1. Type A majority of epidemics
   2. Anti-phagocytic
B. Endotoxin involved in disease (Waterhouse-Frederichsen syndrome)

II. Epidemiology

A. Man is only reservoir - up to 30% carriers
B. Disease appears sporadically or in epidemics in military personnel

The major virulence factors of the

meningococcus are

A. endotoxin

B. IgA protease

C. capsular carbohydrate

D. all of the above

E. A and C only

  (answer at bottom)

III. Pathogenesis

A. gain access to nasopharynx
B. Pili affect adherence
C. local inflammatory rx - organism produces IgA1 protease
D. bacteremia $\rightarrow$ meningitis or meningococcemia
E. result in metastatic lesions in skin (causes purpuric rash), joints, ears, lungs, adrenals, etc.
F. fulminating cases - acute adrenal insufficiency (Waterhouse-Friderichsen syndrome) associated with hemorrhagic necrosis of both adrenal glands

Meningococci adhere to host cells by

means of pili/capsule.

  (answer = D)

NEISSERIA GONORRHOEAE

I. Antigenic Structure

  A. K antigen - cell wall polysaccharide
     lost on subculture: I-IV related
     to virulence and colony morphology;
     I and II are virulent, contain pili
     and are leukocyte associated).
  B. This variability has confounded
     efforts at vaccine development.

Gonococci adhere to host cells by means of pili/capsules.

II. Pathogenicity

  A. Enter through mucous membrane of
     genitourinary tract.
  B. Penetrate between columnar epi-
     thelial cell. In subepithelial
     tissue cause acute inflammatory
     response resulting in purulent yellow
     urethral or vaginal discharge.
  C. Pili responsible for adherence to
     cell membranes and survival within
     PMNs.
  D. Organisms elaborate a protease which
     cleaves IgA1 at the hinge region of
     the H chain.

One of the most serious complications of gonorrhea is PID, which stands for

_____.

III. Symptomatology

  A. Male
   1. incubation period - 2-8 days
   2. frequent, urgent, painful urination
   3. mucopurulent discharge
  B. Female
   1. commonly asymptomatic
   2. urethritis
   3. may involve fallopian tubes; may
      cause pelvic inflammatory disease,
      salpingitis.
  C. Culture is required to confirm
     diagnosis in both males and females

The drug of choice for penicillinase producing N. gonorrhoeae is

_____.

IV. Diseases Other Than Gonorrhea

  A. Arthritis via hematogenous route
  B. Ophthalmia neonatorum acquired
     passing through birth canal

V. Therapy

  A. Penicillin = drug of choice
  B. Spectinomycin for PPNG (Penicillinase
     producing Neisseria gonorrhoeae)

GRAM POSITIVE RODS

BACILLUS ANTHRACIS

I. Pathogenicity of Anthrax
 A. Spore is infectious particle
 B. Penicillin = drug of choice
 C. Three routes of infection
  1. cutaneous (puncture); disease = malignant pustule
  2. ingestion
  3. inhalation (woolsorter's disease)
 D. Virulence
  1. d-polyglutamic acid capsule (anti-phagocytic)
  2. Tri-molecular toxin
  a. Edema factor = adenylate cyclase
  b. Protective antigen - binds to host cell membrane
  c. Lethal factor

The antiphagocytic capsule of

B. anthracis is composed of

_____.

CLOSTRIDIUM GENUS

I. Gas Gangrene: complex infection by anaerobic bacteria

 A. Organisms involved
  1. Clostridium perfringens type, A,D,F
  2. Clostridium novyi
  3. Clostridium septicum

 B. Pathogenicity
  1. Any wound contaminated with dirt has potential for gas gangrene infection due to low redox potential of traumatized tissue.
  2. Toxins and enzymes
  a. alpha toxin - lecithinase C
  b. collagenase, hyaluronidase
  c. hemolysin
  d. enterotoxin = food poisoning

 C. Treatment
  1. antiserum
  2. debridement of wound
  3. hypochlorite or H_2O_2
  4. hyperbaric oxygen
  5. penicillin, tetracycline

The spore is the infectious particle in

all of the following diseases except:

A. tetanus

B. anthrax

C. gas gangrene

D. botulism

  (answer at bottom)

(the best answer to the question above is D, although infant botulism is spore-mediated)

157

II. <u>Tetanus</u> – organism involved –
<u>Clostridium</u> <u>tetani</u>

A. Toxin
1. Tetanus toxin – B chain binds
to cell; A chain is the toxic
moeity.
a. acts at synaptic junction of
specific interneurons to block
inhibitory pathways in anterior
horn cells.
2. Toxoid=prophylaxis; antitoxin=
therapy; single antigenic type

B. <u>Pathogenesis</u>
1. Deep wound and inflammatory response
2. Anaerobic conditions
3. Very limited infection: disease is
an intoxication
4. Toxin production locally; spread
through body intraaxonally
5. Causes spastic paralysis;
opisthotonus.

III. <u>Botulism</u>–organism involved –
Clostridium botulinum

A. <u>Pathogenicity</u>
1. Potent neurotoxin–H chain binds to
cell; L chain is toxic moiety.
a. 8 serologic types–A, B, and E
most common in man.
b. protein, heat labile, resistant
to gastric acidity and
proteolysis; ingested as
prototoxin.
c. mechanism of action – interferes
with release of acetylcholine in
the efferent autonomic nervous
system and prevents the transmission of nerve impulses across
the myoneural junction.

IV. Pseudomembranous enterocolitis
Organism involved = <u>Clostridium</u>
<u>difficile</u>
A. Clindamycin oral therapy is involved
as a precipitating factor. It de-
presses anaerobic gut flora which
allows C. difficile to grow.
B. Vancomycin is the drug of choice.

Tetanus toxin interferes with

_____

_____

_____.

Botulinum toxin interferes with

_____

_____

_____.

The drug of choice for <u>C</u>. <u>difficile</u>

enterocolitis is _____.

158

CORYNEBACTERIA

I. <u>Diphtheria</u> causative agent –
   <u>Corynebacterium</u> <u>diphtheriae</u>;
   diphtheroids = normal flora

A. <u>Diphtheria</u> <u>toxin</u>
   1. Protein of 65-70,000 daltons
   2. Production of toxin
      a. requires the presence of beta
         phage, and low iron content
      b. toxin is a phage-coded protein
         (lysogenic conversion)
   3. Mechanism of action
      a. Fragment B – attaches to cell
         membrane
      b. Fragment A – inhibits protein
         biosynthesis by inhibiting the
         transferase II enzyme, Elongation
         Factor 2, by ADP ribosylation.

B. Disease is due to toxemia. No
   bacteria are found in the blood,
   therefore, the therapy of choice is
   antitoxin, not antibiotics. Prophylactic toxoid stimulates the production of antitoxin.

C. Pseudomembrane that forms in the
   throat is composed of fibrin, PMNs,
   dead tissue cells and bacteria. It
   may break free from the underlying
   epithelium and close off the airway,
   causing suffocation.

D. Diagnosis
   1. Observe Gram + pleomorphic rods
      in palisade arrangement in stain
      of swab of pseudomembrane.
   2. Culture organism on Blood agar,
      Loeffler's or tellurite agars.
   3. Demonstrate metachromatic nature
      of organism.
   4. Prove toxigenicity of organism.
      This is the definitive step; must
      use antitoxin as specificity
      control.

LISTERIA MONOCYTOGENES

   <u>L</u>. <u>monocytogenes</u> – cousin of <u>C</u>.
   <u>diphtheria</u> – but is motile at 24 C.
   A. Causes 10% of neonatal meningitis
      (normal vaginal flora).
   B. Cell wall lipid induces monocytosis.

Diphtheria toxin inhibits protein

synthesis by _____

_____

_____.

Therapy of choice for diphtheria is

_____

_____.

Elongation factor 2 is ADP-ribosylated
by diphtheria toxin. The prokaryotic
translocation factor EF-G is not. This
specificity is due to the presence in
eukaryotic EF-2 of a unique residue,
diphthamide, which is a modified
histidine side chain in the protein
which is the site of ADP-ribose
attachment.

The most common listerial infection
in adults is meningitis; endocarditis
and septicemia may also occur.

159

ACID FAST BACILLI

I. Mycobacterioses

A. Organisms
   1. Mycobacterium tuberculosis (facul-
      tative intracellular parasite)
   2. Mycobacterium leprae (obligate
      intracellular parasite)
   3. Atypical mycobacteria e.g., M.
      kansasi, M. avium intracellulare
   4. BCG = bacille Calmette Guerin;
      a. attenuated M. tuberculosis
         (bovine strain)
      b. vaccine vs. tuberculosis

B. Acid fast due to high lipid content
   (mycolic acids) of cell wall

C. Growth - most are slow growers (M.
   tuberculosis = 3-6 weeks); obligate
   aerobes

D. Toxic product = Cord Factor (trehalose
   6,6 dimycolate) and sulfatides; blocks
   production of toxic oxygen metabolites

E. Cell wall is rich in lipids, (e.g.,
   wax D); resistant to acids, alkali,
   and chemical disinfectants

F. Epidemiology

   1. M. tuberculosis
      a. Man to man or animal to man
         transfer by ingestion, contact,
         or aerosol
   2. Atypical mycobacteria
      a. No man to man transfer
      b. Probable source in soil and water
      c. Portal of entry is upper respir-
         atory tract, or through the skin
      d. M. avium occurs in AIDS patients
   3. M. leprae
      a. Man is major host; agent has
         also been cultured in armadillo
      b. Transmission by prolonged
         contact

G. Diagnosis
   1. Observe acid fast rods in tissue
   2. Culture (except M. leprae)
   3. Niacin test - M. tb = positive,
      atypicals = negative

M. tuberculosis is

A. Acid fast

B. Gram positive

C. Both

D. Neither

(Answer at bottom)

Niacin production is a valuable

laboratory test in the identification of

A. M. tuberculosis

B. M. leprae

C. Both

D. Neither

(answer at bottom)

(answer = C)
(answer = A)

160

H. Treatment

  1. First Line Drugs (atypicals may be
     resistant)
     a. Isoniazid (INH) and PAS
     b. Streptomycin and PAS
     c. Rifampin and ethambutol
     d. INH alone for skin test converters

  2. Second Line Drugs
     a. Ethionamide
     b. Cycloserine
     c. Pyrazinamide

Leprosy

  1. Etiologic agent: M. leprae (Hansen's
     bacillus)

  2. Two types of disease
     a. lepromatous (nodular skin lesions
        with abundant acid fast bacilli;
        lepromin negative)
     b. tuberculoid (anaesthetic macular
        skin lesions with very few acid fast
        bacilli; lepromin positive)

  3. Transmission is by direct contact

  4. Skin testing - lepromin - extract of
     lepromatous nodules

  5. Chemotherapy with DAPSONE

II. Actinomyces israelii

  A. not acid fast

  B. obligate anaerobe; normal oral
     flora

  C. lumpy jaw; cervicofacial abscess
     with "sulfur granule" exudate

  III. Nocardia asteroides

  A. Weakly acid fast

  B. aerobe; soil organism

  C. pulmonary disease in immuno-
     depressed patients; skin and
     subcutaneous infections via
     trauma

First line drugs for tuberculosis include

1. _____

2. _____

3. _____

4. _____

5. _____

Drug of choice for Hansen's bacillus

_____.

Etiologic agent associated with lumpy

jaw is _____.

161

GRAM NEGATIVE RODS

I. Characteristics of interest

A. Some produce exotoxins
B. Enterobacteriaceae are oxidase negative
C. All contain endotoxin
   1. component of cell wall; lipopoly-saccharide (lipid A = toxic part)
   2. pyrogenic; induces release of endogenous pyrogen (interleukin 1) which acts on hypothalamus
   3. B cell mitogen; weakly antigenic
   4. activation of alternate pathway of complement
   5. may trigger disseminated intra-vascular coagulation
D. Eosin Methylene Blue (EMB) agar is useful in isolating enteric organisms

The outer membrane of Gram negative bacteria contains a potent toxin, LPS, which stands for _____.

The toxic moiety is _____.

EMB is a selective/differential/both medium used to purify _____ from mixed flora specimens (e.g. feces).

ESCHERICHIA COLI

I. Diseases

A. Most common cause of urinary tract infections (cystitis, pyelonephritis of pregnancy); 10^5/ml in urine suggests etiology of cystitis
B. Neonatal meningitis: especially during 1st 2 months (with Gp. B strep); ascending infection occurs in utero or organisms are acquired during birth process
C. Epidemic childhood diarrhea common in developing countries
D. Traveler's diarrhea

Diseases produced by E. coli include

1. _____
2. _____
3. _____
4. _____

II. Immunologic Considerations
A. O Antigens - (somatic)
B. H Antigens - (flagellar)
C. K Antigens - (capsule)

III. Products Associated with Disease
A. Adherence pili
B. Endotoxin
C. 2 enterotoxins, 1 is heat stable (↑ quanyl cyclase), the other 1 heat labile, (↑ adenyl cyclase)

Heat labile toxin structure is A-B5: A is an enzyme that ADP ribosylates an adenylate cyclase regulatory protein, increasing cAMP in the enterocyte and causing secretory diarrhea; B binds to GM-1 ganglio-side in the enterocyte membrane.

IV. Therapy
A. Systemic diseases = aminoglycosides
B. Cystitis = sulfonamides, nalidixic acid
C. Diarrhea = trimethoprim + sulfamethoxazole

KLEBSIELLA

I. Diseases Caused by K. pneumoniae

A. Normal flora in 5% of population
B. Important in elderly compromised by major surgical or medical problems and in alcoholics
C. Pneumonia - bronchitis, bronchiectasis. Necrosis accompanied by cavitation and fibrosis
D. Virulence factor = anti-phagocytic capsular polysaccharide
E. Drug of choice = aminoglycosides

SALMONELLA

I. General Characteristics

A. Non-lactose fermenters, Acid and gas from glucose
B. All motile, several species H_2S+

II. Immunology

A. O=somatic antigen and H=flagellar antigen
B. Vi (virulence) antigen--found on S. typhi
C. LPS=endotoxin=major virulence factor
D. Iron binding siderophores (enterochelins) = important for growth

III. Types of Diseases (Salmonelloses)

A. Enteric fevers
B. Septicemia --suppurative lesions; prototype = typhoid fever
C. Gastroenteritis from contaminated food, poultry, poultry products like eggs, etc: an infection, not an intoxication; incubation period = 12-24 hrs
D. Treatment=chloramphenicol, ampicillin

IV. Three species = typhi, cholerae-suis and enteritidis

A. Typhi is restricted to humans, the others are zoonotic
B. Just one organism in each of the first two
C. All of the "old" species are now serotypes of enteritidis

Septicemia occurs commonly in infection with

A. S. typhi

B. S. enteriditis

C. S. cholerae-suis

D. All of the above

E. A and C only

(answer at bottom of page)

(answer = E)

163

SHIGELLA

I. General Characteristics
A. Non-lactose fermenter
B. Differentiated from Salmonella by:
1. acid only from carbohydrates
2. no hydrogen sulfide
3. non-motile (no H antigens)
C. Organisms invade epithelial cells
D. Disease = high fever, bloody diarrhea; local infection
E. Treat with trimethoprim/sulfa

II. Antigenic sutructure
A. Grouping is based on major cell wall carbohydrate antigens (O)

III. Toxic Metabolites
A. All have endotoxin
B. Sh. dysenteriae produces an heat labile A-B5 enterotoxin
1. effects the colon, not the ileum
2. inhibits protein synthesis by reaction with 60S ribosome

VIBRIO CHOLERAE

I. General Characteristics
A. Gram negative, comma shaped
B. Motile
C. Destroyed by heat and disinfectants

II. Pathogenicity due to
A. Enterotoxin (choleragen) stimulates adenyl cyclase and increases intracellular cAMP. Increases the secretion of Cl, HCO_3 and H_2O.
1. A subunit ADP-ribosylates a GTPase (ala diphtheria toxin) thereby blocking its control of adenylate cyclase.
2. B subunit binds to GM-1 ganglioside of epithelial cells.
B. Adherence to the gut epithelium in the jejunum and ileum; local infection.
C. Motility is related to adherence; motile strains adhere

III. Related organisms
A. V. parahemolyticus causes diarrheal disease; source is shellfish
B. V. vulnificus causes diarrheal disease as well as septicemia and wound infections; source is seawater

V. cholerae, cont.

IV. Disease
A. Found only n man; fecal-oral route of transmission
B. Nausea, marked dehydration
C. Rice-water stools and mucus with 20 liters of liquid lost per day
D. Local infection confined to the small intestine - no bacteremia
E. Treatment is supportive with fluids and electrolytes

V. Immunity
A. Due to antibody to microbial cell wall plus antitoxin against the enterotoxin

---

Cholera toxin has an A-B5 structure. A is an enzyme that ADP ribosylates an adenylate cyclase regulatory protein, increases cAMP in the cell, and causes watery diarrhea; B binds to a cell membrane GM-1 ganglioside.

CAMPYLOBACTER JEJUNI

A. This organism, related to V. cholerae morphologically and physiologically, is probably the most common bacterial cause of pediatric diarrhea in the US
B. Symptoms = fever, bloody diarrhea and abdominal pain.
C. Mucosal damage (bloody diarrhea) in small and large intestine.
D. Produces a cytotoxin.

HELICOBACTER PYLORI

A. Cause of peptic ulcers
B. Presence associated with stomach cancer
C. Strongly urease positive

PSEUDOMONAS AERUGINOSA

I. *P. aeruginosa* produces blue-green pus due to production of water soluble pigments (pyocyanin). It is a non-fermenter. It produces oxidase.

II. Clinical significance (as an opportunist)

  A. Hospital acquired infections
    1. Wounds, burns, etc.
    2. Urinary tract via catheter
    3. Respiratory via nebulizers
    4. High rate of multiple drug resistance
    5. Treatment = tobramycin + carbenicillin
  B. Causes pneumonia in cystic fibrosis patients
  C. Produces enterotoxin which causes watery diarrhea
  D. Produces exotoxin A similar to diphtheria (i.e., A and B fragments; interferes with protein synthesis by adenosine ribosylating elongation factor II)
  E. The pseudomonas capsule is composed of Ca++ alginate; it acts as an antiphagocytic virulence factor and is responsible for the micro-colonies seen in lungs of patients with cystic fibrosis.

BACTEROIDES

  I. Gram negative, non-sporeforming, anaerobic rods
  II. The predominant organism in the bowel
 III. Virulence factors
    A. Capsule
    B. Endotoxin is of minor importance
  IV. Diseases = aspiration pneumonia, pulmonary abscesses, septicemia
  V. Treatment = clindamycin

Complete the following table:

	Salmonella	Shigella
acid from lactose	_____	_____
acid from glucose	_____	_____
gas from glucose	_____	_____
hydrogen sulfide	_____	_____
motile	_____	_____

Cholera toxin causes diarrheal disease

by _____.

Major Causes of Wound Infections

Surgical	*Staphylococcus aureus*(1)
Traumatic	Clostridia
Umbilical	C. tetani
Burns	Pseudomonas
Bites	*Pasteurella multocida*

(1) *S. aureus* also seen in burns and umbilical infections

FUSOBACTERIUM

  I. Gram negative anaerobic rod
  II. Normal flora organism
    A. found in the gut and mouth
    B. Observed as cigar-shaped rods
 III. Virulence factors
    A. Endotoxin
    B. Synergistic growth with other bacteria
  IV. Diseases = abscesses, synergistic gangrene, periodontitis, Vincent's angina (trench mouth, acute necrotizing ulcerative gingivitis)
  V. Treatment = clindamycin

GRAM NEGATIVE RESPIRATORY PATHOGENS

HAEMOPHILUS INFLUENZAE

I. <u>Growth factors</u> - requires both:
A. X factor - hematin
B. V factor - NAD

II. <u>Virulence factors</u>
A. Polysaccharide capsule
   1. serotypes a-f (b most common; causes 90% of human disease)
   2. antiphagocytic
B. Endotoxin
C. IgA protease

III. <u>Types of infection</u>
A. Upper respiratory tract-life threatening epiglottitis in infants
B. Lower respiratory tract - pneumonia
C. Meningitis in young children (2-60 months)
D. All of the above are caused by encapsulated strains; non-encapsulated variants produce localized infections such as otitis media.

IV. <u>Culture</u> - growth in presence of X and V factors = Satellite phenomenon

V. <u>Therapy</u> - Chloramphenicol and ampicillin

VI. <u>Prevention</u> - vaccine of type b capsule alone or coupled to carrier proteins such as tetanus toxoid or outer membrane proteins of <u>N</u>. <u>meningitidis</u>

BORDETELLA PERTUSSIS

I. <u>Growth</u>
A. Cultured by cough plate or with pernasal swab
B. Require Bordet-Gengou medium
C. Colonize ciliated epithelial cells of respiratory tract; non-invading

II. <u>Epidemiology of whooping cough</u>
A. Highly contagious disease of humans
   1. 50% of cases are under 4 years old
   2. 67% of deaths are under 1 year
B. Antibodies to <u>B</u>. <u>pertussis</u> do not cross the placental barrier so newborns are completely unprotected.

Most cases of <u>H</u>. <u>influenzae</u> meningitis in young children are due to capsular type _____; non-encapsulated strains are associated with _____.

Cousins of <u>H</u>. <u>influenzae</u> cause:

Disease	Haemophilus species
Pink eye	_____
Soft chancre	_____

(answers on next page)

The drugs of choice for <u>H</u>. <u>influenzae</u> meningitis include _____ and _____.

166

III. Pathogenicity

A. Three stages of whooping cough
   1. Catarrhal stage
   2. Spasmodic (Paroxysmal) stage
   3. Convalescent stage
B. Toxic Products
   1. Carbohydrate capsule
   2. Pilus; adherence organelle
   3. Lipopolysaccharide endotoxin
   4. Pertussis exotoxin; responsible for
      lymphocytosis and histamine
      sensitivity
   5. Adenylate cyclase
C. Localized infection

IV. Immunity
A. Single antigenic type
B. Killed cell vaccine available
   (opsonic immunity)
C. New acellular vaccine composed of 2
   hemagglutinins being developed
   1. fimbrial HA (adherence pilus)
   2. pertussis toxin HA
D. Excellent convalescent immunity

LEGIONELLA PNEUMOPHILA

I. Cause of nosocomial pneumonia
   acquired from the environment,
   e.g., water cooled, air
   conditioning units); not man to man
II. Fastidious Gram negative rod
III. Facultative intracellular parasite
IV. Cell mediated immunity important

Answers to "Cousins" question
   Pink eye = H. aegyptius

   Soft chancre = H. ducreyi

Vaccine induced immunity in whooping
cough is antitoxic/opsonic.

MYCOPLASMA PNEUMONIAE

I. Similar to Protoplasts, Spheroplasts
   and L-forms of Bacteria

   A. Protoplasts and spheroplasts are
      laboratory-induced forms of bacteria
      which contain little or no cell wall;
      induced by penicillin or lysozyme.
   B. Drug of choice = tetracyclines or
      erythromycin
   C. Pathogenesis = organisms attach to
      host cell membrane's sialic acid
      residues via a neuraminidase-like
      receptor. There is no tissue
      invasion, but the production of toxic
      metabolites such as H_2O_2 cause damage
      locally.
   D. Highly pleomorphic organisms without a
      cell wall
   E. Require cholesterol for growth; genus
      Acholeplasma do not

Mycoplasma, protoplasts and spheroplasts

all lack _____

_____ and

are resistant to _____

antibiotics.

III. Disease = primary atypical pneumonia (PAP)

IV. Characteristics of PAP

   A. Non-productive cough
   B. Minimal physical findings; may be
      myalgia, no pleuritic chest pain
   C. Usually normal white blood cell
      count; few polymorphonuclear leuko-
      cytes in sputum
   D. X-ray findings show pulmonary in-
      volvement out of proportion to
      physical findings
   E. Etiologic agents; M. pneumoniae,
      Chlamydia psittaci, Coxiella
      burnetti, adenovirus, respiratory
      syncytical virus, influenza virus,
      parainfluenza virus
   F. Histopathology is of an interstitial
      pneumonia with a mononuclear cell
      infiltrate and very little exudate
      into the alveolar space
   G. Disease caused by Mycoplasma, psitta-
      cosis and Q fever can be treated with
      tetracycline. Other etiologies of
      PAP will not respond to antibiotic
      therapy

Etiologies of primary atypical pneumonia
include:

1. _____

2. _____

3. _____

4. _____

5. _____

168

V. Laboratory Diagnosis of M. pneumoniae

A. Cultures
1. Special media required for isolation; colonies are beta hemolytic
2. Growth requires 1-2 weeks

B. Serology
1. Non-specific
a. Cold hemagglutinins
b. Streptococcus MG agglutinins
2. Specific
a. Dye reduction inhibition test
b. Immunofluorescence
c. Complement fixation

UREAPLASMA

I. Very similar to mycoplasma, but hydrolyze urea

II. Produce extremely tiny colonies (less than 20 microns) hence also called T strains (T=tiny)
   adults
III. Etiology implicated in non-gonococcal urethritis

MOST COMMON CAUSES OF PNEUMONIA	
Age	Microorganism
0 - 1 month	E. coli Group B streptococci
1 - 6 months	Chlamydia Respiratory Syncytial virus (RSV)
1/2 - 5 years	Parainfluenza virus
5 - 15 years	Mycoplasma Influenza virus
16 - 30 years	Mycoplasma
Over 30 years	Streptococcus pneumoniae
Debilitated	Klebsiella pneumoniae

OPPORTUNISTIC PATHOGENS

Source	Microorganism
Normal Flora[1]	Candida Staphylococcus Actinomyces Pneumocystis
Environment	Klebsiella Escherichia Enterobacter Serratia Pseudomonas Legionella Aspergillus Phycomyces

1. Other normal flora may be pathogenic when introduced into normally sterile areas ex. PID with Bacteriodes, aspiration pneumonia with oral flora, peritonitis with gut flora.

GENERALIZED GRAM NEGATIVE PATHOGENS

ALL 3 ARE: FACULTATIVE INTRACELLULAR
            PARASITES
       : ZOONOSES
       : TREATMENT = STREPTOMYCIN

YERSINIA PESTIS

I. Epidemiology of plague

  A. Disease of animals (rodents)
     transmitted to man by
     1. rat fleas (bubonic plague)
     2. direct contact with infected
       animals
  B. Man to man transmission by
     1. human fleas (bubonic)
     2. direct contact - droplet infection
       (pneumonic)
  C. Most cases occur in rural populations
     in contact with wild animals
     (sylvatic)

II. V and W antigens - associated with
     virulence, as is capsular polysacchar-
     ide (F I)

III. Yersinia enterocolitica
  A. Human gastroenteritis with fever,
     diarrhea and cramps, usually in
     children
  B. Produces an enterotoxin similar to E.
     coli heat stable toxin; I quanyl
     cyclase

FRANCISELLA TULARENSIS

I. Epidemiology of tularemia

  A. Disease of rodents (rabbits and
     squirrels)
  B. Transmitted to man by contact with
     infected animal, by tick bites, and
     by ingestion of water

II. Two types of disease

  A. Ulceroglandular
  B. Typhoidal (must be distinguished from
     typhoid fever)

(answers = C and E)

Y. pestis is a

  A. facultative intracellular parasite.

  B. zoonotic agent transmitted to may by

     rat fleas.

  C. both

  D. neither

(answer at bottom, left)

F. tularensis is

  A. transmitted to man by infected ticks.

  B. an obligate intracellular parasite.

  C. susceptible to streptomycin.

  D. all of the above.

  E. A and C only.

(answer at left)

GARDNERELLA VAGINALIS

  I. normal vaginal flora
 II. causes vaginitis with fishy
     odoriferous discharge; may be mixed
     infection
III. Diagnosis = clue cells; epithelium
     adherent coccobacilli
 IV. treat = metronidazole (same for
     trichomonas)

170

BRUCELLA

I. Introduction

A. Three species
   1. Brucella suis - swine
   2. Brucella melitensis - goats, sheep
   3. Brucella abortus - cattle

II. Tissue trophism - B. abortus

A. Infection in animals usually limited
   to placenta due to high concentration
   of erythritol
   1. Abortion
   2. Infection of supramammary lymph
      nodes and spillage of organisms into
      milk
B. In man infection is usually generalized

B. abortus is a cause of abortion in

cattle due to _____

_____

_____.

III. Clinical types of Brucella
     infections

A. Intermittent-high fever rising to
   101-104 C; night sweats
B. Chronic-CNS abnormalities seen
C. Undulant-step wise increases in
   temperature over a period of days
D. Malignant - sustained high temperature, extreme hyperpyrexia before
   death

IV. Pathogenicity

A. Organisms are continually phago-
   cytosed by the reticuloendothelial
   system, then released into the blood
   stream
B. Virulent organisms resist intracellular killing

Treatment of brucellosis involves _____

_____

_____

_____.

V. Treatment

A. Combination of streptomycin and
   tetracycline recommended
B. Chronic nature of the infection may
   necessitate prolonged period of
   therapy

171

SPIROCHETES

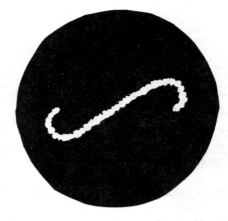

I. Introduction
  A. Organisms
   1. Genus <u>Borrelia</u>
   2. Genus <u>Leptospira</u>
   3. Genus <u>Treponema</u>
  B. Morphology and Growth

Genus	Morphology	Oxygen Requirements
<u>Borrelia</u>	Long with loose spirals	micro-aerophilic
<u>Leptospira</u>	Fine, tight spirals with hooked ends	aerobes
<u>Treponema</u>	Short with tight spirals	anaerobes

The organism shown above most likely

A. can grow in the presence of oxygen.

B. causes relapsing fever.

C. causes sexually transmitted diseases.

D. causes Lyme disease.

E. causes acute necrotizing ulcerative gingivitis.

(answer below)

LEPTOSPIRA

A. Organism involved - <u>L</u>. <u>interrogans</u>
B. Description of disease process
   1. Fever with jaundice
   2. Infection of kidney and liver; acute hemorrhagic hepatitis
C. Epidemiology
   1. Parasites of wild and domesticated animals
   2. Infection by contact with urine from infected animals or water contaminated with urine

BORRELIA

A. Organisms involved
   1. <u>B</u>. <u>burgdorferi</u> - Lyme disease
   2. <u>B</u>. <u>recurrentis</u> - relapsing fever
B. Reservoir and Transmission
   1. Organism is perpetuated by tick-animal cycle
   2. Maintained in tick by transovarial transmission
   3. Wound created by tick bite is con-taminated with secretions and excretions of tick
   4. Endemic disease
   5. Reservoirs
      a. Relapsing fever = rodents, humans in epidemics
      b. Lyme disease = deer
   6. Vectors (ticks)
      a. Relapsing fever = <u>Ornithodorus</u> spp.
      b. Lyme disease = <u>Ixodes</u> <u>dammani</u>

(answer = A)

C. Description of Relapsing Fever
  1. abrupt onset with chills, fever
     (3-10 days), generalized pain,
     prostration and delirium
  2. free interval of 1-3 weeks followed
     by several relapses; relapses due to
     emergence of new antigenic types
D. Borrelia also seen in Vincent's
   angina, fuso-spirochetal stomatitis;
   acute necrotizing ulcerative
   gingivitis

TREPONEMA PALLIDUM

Stages of syphilis

1. Primary stage
   a. lesion usually appears 10-30 days
      after infection
   b. Hunterian (hard chancre) -
      indolent, indurated ulcer, usually
      single, painless; loaded with
      spirochetes

2. Secondary stage
   a. usually occurs 6-12 weeks after
      chancre
   b. invasion of skin, eyes, blood
      stream, cerebrospinal fluid
   c. ulcerating, necrotic lesions of
      skin (rash), alopecia, numerous
      spirochetes

3. Tertiary stage [months - years later]
   a. gummata of skin, bones, nervous
      system, no organisms seen
   b. cardiovascular and neurosyphilis

4. Congenital syphilis
   a. primary and secondary stages occur
      in utero
   b. child has latent stage upon birth

Serologic diagnosis of syphilis
1. VDRL and RPR
   a. antibody measured (reagin) is not
      specific antibody for T. pallidum

2. FTA-abs (Fluorescent Treponemal
   Antibody-Absorption Test)
   a. Serum contains antibody to organism
   b. Fluorescent labelled antiglobulin
      reacts with Ab fixed to spirochete

The drug of choice for
syphilis is penicillin.
Erythromycin is used in
cases of penicillin
allergy.

ERYTHEMA CHRONICUM MIGRANS

Lyme disease is a condition
of spirochetal etiology which
is characterized by a migrat-
ing erythematous rash that is
usually followed a few weeks
later by migratory poly-
arthritis. The organism is
spread by the bite of ticks.
First described as an epidemic
in Lyme, Conn. The etiologic
agent, Borrelia burgdorferi,
has a tissue tropism similar
to treponemes (i.e., heart,
nerves and bone). Some un-
treated patients develop
cardiac and neurologic
manifestations.

Spirochetes are readily
demonstrated in
primary/secondary/tertiary
syphilis.

BACTERIA, RICKETTSIAE, CHLAMYDIAE AND VIRUSES

CHARACTERISTICS IN COMPARISON

	Characteristic	Bacteria	Rickettsiae & Chlamydiae	Viruses
1.	Obligate intracellular parasite	-	+	+
2.	Growth on lifeless media	+	-	-
3.	Contain both DNA and RNA	+	+	-
4.	Multiple by fission	Binary	Binary & Unequal*	Subunit Assembly
5.	Visible with light microscope	+	+	-
6.	Contains muramic acid in cell wall	+	+	-
7.	Independent metabolic activity	+	+	-
8.	Possess ribosomes	+	+	-
9.	Susceptible to antibacterial antibiotics	+	+	-

*Reticulate bodies multiply and then disintegrate into elementary bodies.

RICKETTSIAE AND CHLAMYDIAE

Properties of the two groups:

1. Considered to be bacteria rather than viruses because they:

   a. Contain both DNA and RNA.
   b. Multiply by binary fission, chlamydia also multiply by unequal fission involving elementary and reticulate bodies.
   c. Contain some metabolically active enzymes.
   d. Contain ribosomes.
   e. Resemble Gram-negative bacteria in that they possess a cell wall with inner and outer membranes.
   f. Are inhibited by antibiotics, e.g., tetracycline.
   g. Are obligate intracellular microorganisms, intermediate in size between large viruses and small bacteria.
   h. Each group has toxic properties associated with the cell. This endotoxin differs from lipopolysaccharide in that it can be detoxified, and is neutralized by type-specific antisera.

2. The two groups differ, in general as follows:

   a. Rickettsiae (R) have an arthropod vector; Chlamydiae (C) do not.
   b. R are transmitted by the bite of the vector; C by droplet or contact.
   c. R diseases involve endothelial lining of blood vessels; C are localized infectious processes (e.g., lungs, eyes)
   d. Tetracycline is the drug of choice for both. Sulfa is contraindicated for R and for psittacosis.
   e. Serodiagnosis of R is by Weil Felix agglutination and C fixation. C diseases are diagnosed by C fixation and neutralization.
   f. R have peptidoglycan in cell wall; C do not.

Bacterial characteristics of Rickettsia include:

1. _____
2. _____
3. _____
4. _____
5. _____
6. _____
7. _____
8. _____

Complete the following Table:

Characteristic	Rickettsia
Disease Transmitted by Vector	
Tissue Tropism	
Drug of Choice	
Serodiagnosis	

175

ETIOLOGY AND EPIDEMIOLOGY OF RICKETTSIAL DISEASE

DISEASES[1]	AGENTS	ARTHROPOD VECTORS[2]	RESERVOIR
Epidemic typhus	R. prowazekii	human louse	Human
Brill's relapsing typhus	R. prowazekii	None	Human
Endemic or murine typhus	R. typhi	rat flea	Rodents
Tsutsugamushi fever (Scrub typhus)	R. tsutsugamushi	chigger mite	Rodents
Rocky Mountain Spotted Fever	R. rickettsii	tick	Dogs rodents
Rickettsialpox	R. akari	mite	Mice
Q fever	Coxiella burnetii	None; human inhalation of dried infectious material, ingestion of contaminated milk	Cattle, sheep, etc.

[1] All except C. burneti invade endothelial cells of vasculature; thrombosis = rash; Treatment = tetracyclines, chloramphenicol

[2] All vectors are infected for life; some (louse & flea) die of disease

CHLAMYDIAL AGENTS

Agent*	Disease	Mode of Transmission
Group A:		
Chlamydia _trachomatis_	Trachoma	Contact with infected human or fresh fomites
	Inclusion conjunctivitis	Passage out birth canal; contact
	Infant pneumonia	Passage out birth canal; contact
	Urethritis	Sex mediated
	Lymphogranuloma venereum; salpingitis	Sex mediated
Group B:		
Chlamydia _psittaci_	Psittacosis	Contact with sick birds and their infectious excreta; inhalation of infectious material from birds.

* Treatment: Group A: Sulfonamides and/or tetracyclines
  Group B: tetracyclines

MEDICAL MYCOLOGY

Agent and Disease	Infectious* Particle	APPEARANCE
Cryptococcus neoformans meningitis	yeast	encapsulated yeast
Candida albicans vulvovaginitis, thrush	yeast; endogenous infection	yeast and pseudohyphae in vivo; add chlamydospores in vitro
Sporothrix schenckii lymphadenitis	microconidia	hyphae: spores in "daisy" clusters (RT)
Blastomyces dermatididis lung & skin	microconidia	hyphae: microconidia (RT) yeast; broadbased bud (37)**
Histoplasma capsulatum lung and RES	microconidia	hyphae: tuberculate macroconidia (RT): intracellular yeast (37)**
Coccidioides immitis lung and brain	arthrospores	hyphae: arthrospores (RT) spherules (37)**
Mucor & Rhizopus spp. Phycomycosis blood vessels and lung	spores	coenocytic hyphae, sporangia
Aspergillus spp. lungs and systemic	spores	septate hyphae and spores

* Only 2 dermatohphytes spread from man to man (M. audouini & T. tonsurans), the rest are environmental or normal flora.   **Dimorphic (37C=yeast, 24C=mold)

ANTIFUNGAL DRUGS

Drug	Agents/Diseases	Mechanism of action
Amphotericin B*	Systemic fungi, e.g. Histo, Cocci, Blasto, Crypto, Aspergillosis	Binds to ergosterol in cell membrane; causes pore formation and cytosol leaks out
Ketokonazole Clotrimazole Miconazole	Most systemics except aspergillosis	Similar to amphotericin B
Flucytosine	Yeasts, Candidiasis Cryptococcosis	Incorporated into RNA and blocks protein sythesis
Potassium iodide	Sporotrichosis	Unknown
Griseofulvin	Dermatophytoses	Interferes with cell division
Tolnaftate	"	Unknown

* Related polyene, Nystatin, is limited to topical use vs Candida

MEDICAL PARASITOLOGY

EPIDEMIOLOGY AND PATHOGENESIS OF
PARASITIC INFECTIONS

TRANSMITTED VIA INGESTION OF OVA

Parasite	Pathogenesis
Enterobius vermicularis	Adults in rectum and colon; Most common parasite of children; anal pruritis.
Ascaris lumbricoides	Adults in small intestine; light infections asympto matic; occasional intestinal obstructions or abnormal migrations of adult in heavy infection.
Toxocara canis	Larvae invade various organs; mark eosinophilia; $\uparrow$ IgE, hepatosplenomegaly, occasionally retinal granuloma due to larval migration.
Trichuris trichiura	Adults in colon and rectum; light infections asymptomatic; heavy infections may cause diarrhea, tenesmus and rectal prolapse.
Taenia solium	Larvae (cysticercus) in all tissues; CNS damage may be serious.
Echinococcus granulosus	Growth of hydatid cyst damages liver or lung.

Complete the Following Table:

Agent	Disease
Taenia	
	Anal pruritis
Echinococcus	
	Visceral larval migrans
Toxoplasma	Disease = Reservoir =
	Muscle pain, ocular edema, eosinophilia
Giardia	
	B12 deficiency and macrocytic anemia
Naegleria	
	Iron deficiency anemia
Strongyloides	

179

TRANSMISSION VIA INGESTION OF CYST

Entamoeba histolytica	Primary ulcers in large intestine; secondary abscess in liver or other organs.
Giardia lamblia	Asymptomatic to protracted diarrhea.
Toxoplasma gondii	Usually asymptomatic in adults; serious CNS damage to fetus if mother infected during pregnancy. Obligate intracellular parasite. Cat reservoir.

TRANSMISSION VIA INGESTION OF LARVAE

Trichinella spiralis	Adults cause GI disturbances; larvae cause muscle pains, ocular edema, eosinophilia.
Taenia saginata	Adult in small intestine may cause vague GI disturbances
Taenia solium	Adult in small intestine may cause vague GI disturbances
Diphylobothrium latum	Vague GI disturbances; rarely vitamin B12 deficiency with macrocytic (pernicious) anemia.

TRANSMISSION VIA LARVAL PENETRATION OF SKIN

Necator americanus or Ancylostoma duodenale	Adults in small intestines; light infections are asymptomatic; heavy infection plus malnutrition causes hypoalbuminemia and iron deficiency anemia.
Strongyloides stercoralis	Adults in small intestinal mucosa; symptoms vary, i.e. asymptomatic, mucoid diarrhea with malabsorption potentially fatal in immunological comprised host (e.g. AIDS) due to autoinfection.

TRANSMISSION VIA CERCARIAL PENETRATION OF SKIN

Schistosoma mansoni or S. japonicum	Granulomatous reactions to eggs deposited in intestinal venules or those trapped in liver or other organs.

TRANSMISSION VIA BITE OF ARTHROPOD VECTOR

Plasmodium vivax, etc. [vector = Anopheles mosquito]	Fever, musculoskeletal pains, severe headache, diarrhea; capillary occlusions in falciparum are especially dangerous.
Onchocerca volvulus [vector = Simulium fly]	Larvae develop into adult worms in subcutaneous tissue; cause formation of tumor-like nodules. Microfilarial forms migrate through eye and may cause blindness.
Wuchereria bancrofti [vector = Anopheles mosquito]	Larva develop into adults in lymphatics. Host's immediate and delayed allergic responses to these causes lymphadenitis which may develop to elephantiasis.
Leishmania [vector = sandflies]	Hyperplasia of cells of the RES. May be localized cutaneous ulcer or severe systemic disease.
Trypanosoma	T. cruzi = Chagas' disease [vector = reduviid bugs] T. gambiense = African sleeping sickness [vector = tsetse fly]

TRANSMISSION VIA DIRECT CONTACT AND/OR INVASION

Trichomonas vaginalis	Local, non-fatal disease; usually symptomatic in females as vaginitis
Naegleria fowleri	Travel up olfactory to brain; cause amebic meningoencephalitis.

PARASITE CHEMOTHERAPY

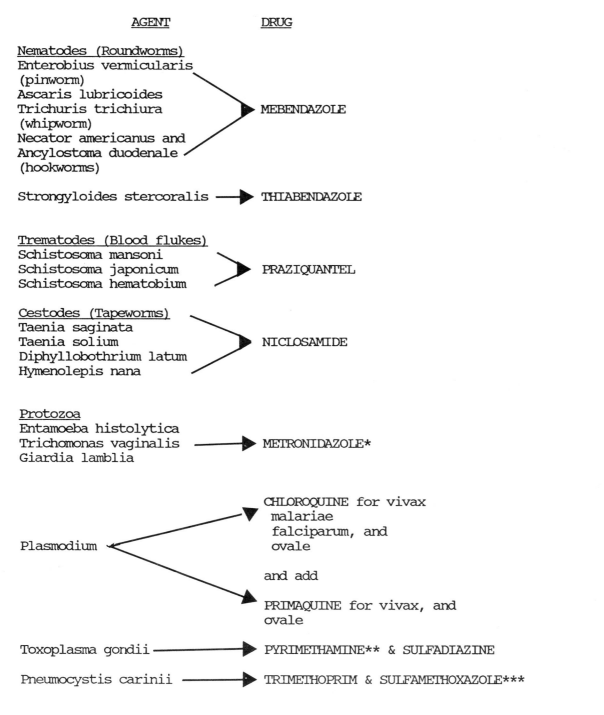

AGENT   **DRUG**

Nematodes (Roundworms)
Enterobius vermicularis
(pinworm)
Ascaris lubricoides
Trichuris trichiura
(whipworm)   MEBENDAZOLE
Necator americanus and
Ancylostoma duodenale
(hookworms)

Strongyloides stercoralis ——▶ THIABENDAZOLE

Trematodes (Blood flukes)
Schistosoma mansoni
Schistosoma japonicum   PRAZIQUANTEL
Schistosoma hematobium

Cestodes (Tapeworms)
Taenia saginata
Taenia solium   NICLOSAMIDE
Diphyllobothrium latum
Hymenolepis nana

Protozoa
Entamoeba histolytica
Trichomonas vaginalis ——▶ METRONIDAZOLE*
Giardia lamblia

                              CHLOROQUINE for vivax
                                malariae
                                falciparum, and
                                ovale
Plasmodium ◀
                              and add

                              PRIMAQUINE for vivax, and
                                ovale

Toxoplasma gondii ——▶ PYRIMETHAMINE** & SULFADIAZINE

Pneumocystis carinii ——▶ TRIMETHOPRIM & SULFAMETHOXAZOLE***

  * also useful vs. anaerobes, Gardnerella, quinacrine also used vs. Giardia
 ** Teratogenic - do not use in first trimester
*** Pentamidine is used in patients who find T/S toxic

181

MECHANISMS OF ACTION OF ANTIPARASITIC DRUGS

Sulfonamides	Blocks conversion of PABA to dihydrofolic acid
Trimethoprim	Inhibits dihydrofolate reductase
Mebendazole	Blocks glucose uptake
Thiabendazole	Inhibits fumarate reductase
Praziquantel	Induces loss of Ca++ with muscular spasms in parasite
Niclosamide	Uncouples phosphorylation
Metronidazole	Alkylation of DNA
Quinine drugs	Intercalates into dsDNA of blocks DNA synthesis

DNA VIRUSES

HERPES VIRUSES

Properties of the group
Enveloped dsDNA viruses with
cubic symmetry. Multiply
in the nucleus

Herpes simplex serotypes 1 & 2

Epidemiology
Man is the only host; spread
by close contact.

Clinical features

Primary disease
Vesicular lesions of the mouth,
lips, etc seen in young children
Recurrent disease
The herpes viruses have a great
propensity to develop **latent
infections** (i.e., the disease
disappears but the virus stays
hence recrudescence of disease
can occur later). Cold sores
(**stomatitis**) are vesicular
lesions which may be triggered by
fever, trauma, menses, stress, etc.
Neonatal disease
A rare but highly fatal infection
of the neonate characterized high
fever, jaundice and encephalitis.
Other diseases
The most common are **genital** sores
particularly with the **type 2** virus;
keratitis and **encephalitis** are
more serious but less common.
Herpetic whitlow is an infection
of the end of the finger. It occurs
commonly in dental professionals.

Treatment

Acyclovir is a very effective
drug; Ara C is also useful as are
idoxuridine and trifluorothymidine

Diagnosis

Culture or **immunofluorescence** stain
or Tzanck stain to see multinucleate
cells with intranuclear inclusions

Herpes viruses

1. are DNA/RNA

2. are single/double stranded

3. are naked/enveloped

4. multiply in the

    nucleus/cytoplasm

5. have helical/cubic

    symmetry

Drugs that are effective

against Herpes simplex include

1. _____

2. _____

3. _____

Most cases of genital herpes

are caused by type 1/2.

The herpes infection at the

ends of fingers and around

nails is called _____

_____. It is an

occupational disease of

_____.

Varicella (chickenpox or Herpes zoster)

Serotype

There is only one serotype of the varicella-zoster virus

Epidemiology
1. Man is the natural host
2. The overall incidence of infection is very high.
3. Transmission probably follows inhalation of infective aerosols, or direct skin contact

Clinical features
1. The onset is sudden, with a rash progressing from macules to papules to vesicles. Pustules do not develop; there is no scarring
2. The lesions appear in successive crops over 3 to 4 days
3. The lesions are distributed chiefly on the trunk and face

Zoster (Herpes zoster or shingles)

Epidemiology

This disease occurs chiefly in adults, most of whom give a history of having had varicella. Infection is communicable from as early as 5 days before to one week after the rash first appears

Pathogenesis

The virus probably persists in cells of the root ganglia after an attack of varicella, and is activated later with a resultant inflammatory reaction along the nerve followed by destruction of the epithelial cells served by that nerve

Clinical features
1. Erythematous maculopapular lesions develop, and on the trunk these have a band-like distribution

2. A disseminated form of disease is sometimes seen in patients who have received immunosuppressive therapy or radiotherapy

Herpes zoster causes

A. chicken pox

B. cold sores

C. shingles

D. all of the above

E. A and C only

(answer at bottom)

Positive heterophile hemagglutinating antibodies are seen in infectious mononucleosis caused by

A. Cytomegalovirus

B. Epstein-Barr virus

C. Both

D. Neither

[see next page for answer]

[answer = E]

184

Infectious mononucleosis

Etiologic agent   (Epstein-Barr)
herpesvirus.
Epidemiology
1. Man is the natural host
2. Infection is most common in young
   adults
3. Incidence of infection is high
4. Mode of transmission; inhalation
   of infective aerosols during
   close personal association
5. Viruses associated with Burkitt's
   lymphoma and nasopharyngeal carcinoma
Serodiagnosis
  The heterophile agglutination test
detects a IgM hemagglutinin vs sheep RBC

Cytomegalic inclusion disease

Etiologic agent
Cytomegalovirus; multiple serotypes
are known
Epidemiology
   1. Man is the only known natural host
   2. The virus can be transmitted across
      the placenta and cause congenital
      infection. The mode of postnatal
      transmission is unclear, but the
      virus is excreted in saliva, semen,
      milk and urine
Clinical features
1. Intrauterine infections may cause
   death of the fetus, or result in congenital disease which is frequently
   fatal. In those who survive, hepato-
   splenomegaly with jaundice, blood
   dyscrasias, cerebral calcification,
   mental retardation, mircocephaly and
   chorioretinitis are common sequelae
2. Postnatal infections are usually
   symptomless in infants and children,
   but occasionally hepatitis, pneumonitis or acquired hemolytic anemia
   develop
3. In patients with malignancies, AIDS,
   or those receiving immunosuppressive
   therapy, hepatitis, pneumonitis,
   infectious mononucleosis-like disease
   (with negative hetrophile),pneumonia,
   or even generalized disease may
   develop, possible resulting from the
   activation of latent virus

> Burkitt's lymphoma occurs in young black
> males in Central Africa. The disease is
> the result of the translocation of a
> piece of chromosome 8 which contains an
> oncogene (c-myc) to the D-J joining
> region or an S switch region in the
> immunoglobulin H chain locus of chromo-
> some 14. Apparently this occurs while
> pre-B cell is undergoing rearrangement
> of genes preparatory to production of
> antibodies. Once the c-myc oncogene
> is translocated to this genetically
> active site it gets turned on and its
> product, a nuclear binding protein that
> is involved in cell activation, is made
> in abnormally high amounts driving the
> the cell to repeated replications.

Epstein-Barr virus is associated with
what two human malignancies (see Oncogenic Viruses section)?

1. _____

2. _____

> Human Herpes virus 6
> causes sixth disease
> [exanthem subitum]
> ----------------------
> Parvorvirus B19 is
> the cause of fifth
> disease [erythema
> infectiosum]

(answer = B)

185

ADENOVIRUSES

Properties of the group

1. Naked viruses, which have an icosahedral nucleocapsid, contain double-stranded DNA and replicate in the nucleus
2. There are more than 40 human serotypes, some cause tumors in animals

Diseases caused by adenoviruses

A. Pharyngo-conjunctival fever

1. Particularly common in military recruits; in the general population, only about 5% of all respiratory illness is caused by adenoviruses
2. The mode of transmission is via infective aerosols or fresh fomites
3. Bronchitis and pneumonia sometimes occur, the latter usually in infants

B. Epidemic keratoconjunctivitis

1. Associated with serotype 8
2. Outbreaks in certain industries are associated with minor ocular trauma resulting from dusty atmosphere

C. Exanthem

Adenovirus is possibly responsible for a rubelliform rash

D. Hemorrhagic Cystitis

Particularly in children

PARVOVIRUSES

Properties of the group
1. Naked, single stranded DNA

Diseases caused by Parvovirus B19
1. Fifth disease (erythema infectiosum)
   a. primarily a disease of children
   b. in individuals with chronic hemolytic diseases such as sickle cell disease or thalassemia B19 infections can precipitate an acute, sometimes fatal, anemia.

Adenoviruses are

1. DNA/RNA.

2. single/double stranded.

3. naked/enveloped.

4. multiply in the nucleus/cytoplasm.

5. helical/cubic symmetry.

Diseases caused by Parvoviruses include

1. _____

2. _____

3. _____

186

PAPOVAVIRUSES

Properties of the group

Naked viruses, which have an icosahedral
nucleocapsid, contain dsDNA, and
replicate in the nucleus

Papilloma virus
Several serotypes affect humans

Epidemiology

1. Man is the only known host
2. The mode of transmission is presumably
   by direct contact

Pathogenesis and pathology

Replication occurs in the epithelial
cells of the skin, virus causes a benign
neoplasm. Papilloma #16 has a high
association with cervical carcinoma

Clinical features

The common wart - serotypes 1 and 4
cervical carcinoma - serotypes 16 and 18
condyloma acuminatum - serotypes 6 and 11

Polyoma virus

Causes many different malignancies in
several animal species

Vacuolating virus

A simian virus (SV40) causes tumors when
inoculated into newborn animals. Also
transforms cells in culture

JC virus

Has been isolated from immunocompromised
individuals and from the brains of
patients with progressive multifocal
leukoencephalopathy. Most humans have
specific antibody vs. the JC virus

The papovavirus responsible for the

common wart is _____.

The papovavirus associated with

progressive multifocal

leukoencephalopathy is

_____.

Papilloma virus serotype 16 is associated

with

_____.

187

POXVIRUSES

Properties of the group

Complex ellipsoid viruses, which contain
double-stranded DNA, replicate in the
cytoplasm; virion contains many enzymes
(e.g. DNA-dependent RNA polymerase)

Smallpox
Epidemiology

1. Man is the only natural host; disease
   has been eradicated from the planet
2. Smallpox is transmitted by inhalation
   of infective aerosols through
   personal association, or by
   contaminated fomites such as bedding

Treatment

Methisazone, which is of value prophy-
lactically, is also useful in treating
dermal complications following vaccination. It blocks synthesis of certain
viral proteins thus inhibiting viral
replication

Artificially-acquired immunity
Active (vaccination)

Immunization is carried out with live
vaccinia virus

Molluscum contagiosum
Epidemiology

Infection probably occurs through minor
abrasions, and in swimming pools

Clinical features

Multiple discrete benign tumors appear on
the skin anywhere except on the palms and
soles; the lesions last for several
months, and then disappear spontaneously

Poxviruses are

1. DNA/RNA.

2. single/double stranded.

3. naked/enveloped.

4. multiply in the cytoplasm/nucleus.

5. helical/cubic/complex symmetry.

A Poxvirus which causes benign

skin tumors in humans is

_____.

RNA VIRUSES

ORTHOMYXOVIRUSES

Properties of the group
1. Enveloped viruses, helical nucleocapsid, contain 8 distinct segments of
   single-stranded RNA and replicate in
   both nucleus and cytoplasm
2. Orthomyxoviruses cause influenza

Serotypes
1. There are 3 serotypes: A, B and C.
2. Each contains 2 surface antigens (H
   and N):
   a. A hemagglutinin (H) which enables
      the virion to attach to receptors
      on the cell surface
   b. A neuraminidase (N) which
      facilitates the release of progeny
      virus from infected cells
3. The 2 surface antigens of serotypes A
   and B undergo frequent antigenic
   changes (caused by point mutations)
   resulting in antigenic "drift"
4. Antigen "shift" is a much more
   drastic change which is caused by
   reassortment of RNA segments of the
   viral (human or animal) genome
5. All known pandemics have been caused
   by serotype A/B/C influenza virus.
   (answer at bottom, right)

Serodiagnosis

Using the hemagglutination-inhibition
technique, the patient's serum can be
tested for antibody against a particular
strain of virus.

Antiviral therapy

Amantadine hydrochloride (Symmetrel) is
used as a prophylactic drug before or
immediately after exposure to influenza A.
It acts by blocking penetration of the
virus into cells and also blocks uncoating
of the virus.

Artificially-acquired immunity
Induced by egg-derived virusess inactivated
by formalin or by subunit vaccines

Reye's syndrome (encephalopathy and fatty liver) is
associated with type B, and
perhaps also with other
viruses (e.g. chickenpox).
Salicylates may also be
involved in the pathogenesis
of the disease.

Influenza is an ssRNA virus whose genome

is in _____

segments. It agglutinates RBCs through

the action of its _____;

the enzyme _____

facilitates progeny release.

(Pandemics = A)

189

PARAMYXOVIRUSES

Properties of the group

Enveloped viruses, helical nucleocapsid, contain single-stranded RNA, and replicated in the cytoplasm. The measles virus is known to replicate in both nucleus and cytoplasm

Parainfluenzavirus infections

The viruses cause a variety of upper and lower respiratory tract illnesses; cold-like ills, pharyngitis, bronchitis, bronchiolitis and pneumonia. In young children, the viruses are the commonest cause of acute laryngotracheobronchitis (croup)

Respiratory Syncytial Virus (RSV) Infection

1. In the infant, severe necrotizing bronchiolitis can occur; bacterial complications are common
2. RSV is the most common cause of viral pneumonia in infants
3. Reinfection occurs commonly, but is usually mild and confined to the upper respiratory tract, frequently resulting in the common cold syndrome
4. Ribavirin is used in therapy in patients likely to have serious disease and sequelae (e.g., patients with a history of coronary heart disease)

Mumps

1. Sudden onset of swelling of the parotid glands, usually bilateral
2. Submaxillary and sublingual glands may also be involved
3. Inflammation of the testis (orchitis) often occurs in males past puberty, but testicular atrophy or sterility is rare
4. Meningitis is a relatively common complication

Respiratory syncytial virus is the most common cause of _____

_____.

Complications of mumps infection include

1. _____

2. _____

Paramyxovirus infections with agents such as RSV can be treated with _____. This chemotherapeutic is very expensive, hence treatment is limited to patients in which the disease may be life-threatening.

190

Measles

1. Cytopathic effect = multinucleated giant cells with nonspecific cytoplasmic and nuclear inclusions
2. Prodromal signs are photophobia, fever, cough, coryza, conjunctivitis and appearance of Koplik's spots in the mouth
3. Viremia
4. After 3 days, a rash starts on the head and spreads to chest, trunk and limbs in the next day or two; the rash disappears slowly
5. May have a transient depression of cell mediated immune responses
6. Complications are fairly common, and sometimes severe: These include - otitis media and pneumonia
7. Encephalomyelitis: rare, occurs 1 to 2 weeks after the rash, and is associated with a high mortality rate
8. Subacute sclerosing panencephalitis may be a post-infection sequela
9. May be transient depression of cell mediated immunity during infections

Prodromal signs of measles include

1. _____
2. _____
3. _____
4. _____
5. _____

ARENAVIRUSES

Properties of the group

Enveloped RNA viruses
Rodent reservoirs: no vector; disease acquired via contact with rodent urine, etc.

Lymphocytic choriomeningitis

A disease usually manifest as "aseptic" meningitis or a mild influenza-like illness, rarely as a severe encephalomyelitis. The natural host of the virus is the mouse

Lassa fever

Hemorrhagic fever with bradycardia, neurologic manifestations and shock

Complications of measles include

1. _____
2. _____
3. _____
4. _____

191

ARTHROPOD-BORNE VIRAL DISEASES

Classification

1. The arboviruses encompass a heterogenous collection of some 400 viruses
   related only by the epidemiological
   fact that they are arthropod-borne
2. The so-called 'arboviruses' alternate
   between an invertebrate vector and a
   vertebrate reservoir
3. Arboviruses belong to several viral
   families: <u>Togaviridae</u>, <u>Bunyaviridae</u>,
   <u>Reoviridae</u>, <u>Flaviviridae</u> and
   others

Epidemiology

1. The cycle of transmission of these
   viruses is from arthropod to
   vertebrate host and back to arthropod
2. The arthropods involved are commonly
   mosquitoes, but sometimes ticks,
   sandflies and gnats act as vectors
3. The natural hosts, which act as
   reservoirs, include birds, reptiles,
   mammals and, rarely, man

BUNYAVIRUSES

Bunyamwera viruses are enveloped,
spherical viruses with helical symmetry.
They are similar ecologically to the
togaviruses and are arthropod-borne
(arboviruses). The single-stranded RNA
is composed of three segments. The
pathogenesis of disease is similar to the
togaviruses (encephalitis). One group of
this diverse family of viruses which has
been associated with encephalitis in
humans is California viruses, first found
in California and more recently in other
parts of the USA

Arthropod-borne viral diseases belong to
the following viral families

1. _____

2. _____

3. _____

4. _____

There are four major pathogens
in the Parainfluenza group:

1. _____

2. _____

3. _____

4. _____

192

TOGAVIRUSES

Arbovirus encephalitis
Most arboviruses are antigenic groups A or B. They are enveloped ssRNA viruses with (+mRNA) genome

1. These encephalitides in the USA include Venezuelan, Western and Eastern equine viruses
2. The usual reservoir is birds, and the vector is the mosquito
3. Clinical findings include fever, chills, headache, widespread muscular aches, drowsiness, nuchal rigidity, convulsions, paralysis, coma and death. (EEE has 50-70% mortality rate)

FLAVIVIRUSES

Yellow fever
1. The natural host is the monkey, and the vector is the _Aedes_ mosquito; two forms of yellow fever, the urban and the jungle (sylvatic), are recognized
2. In the urban type of yellow fever, man is the main reservoir, and the transmission cycle is man-mosquito-man
3. In the jungle type, the monkey is the main reservoir, and the cycle is monkey-mosquito-monkey with man being infected occasionally
4. The outstanding feature in cases of yellow fever is the extent of damage to liver and kidney in severe cases

Dengue
1. Man is the reservoir for this virus
2. The onset of illness is characterized by fever, chills, headache, conjunctivitis, lymphadenitis, severe pain in the back, muscles and joints ('break-bone fever')
3. Fever often falls, then rises again within a week ("saddleback curve")
4. Dengue hemorrhagic fever is a severe disease with a 10% mortality which occurs in individuals who have passive maternal antibody or have recovered from a previous attack by a different dengue serotype. Virus/antibody complexes form early in the disease; they activate complement with the result of DIC and shock.

Clinical signs of viral encephalitis include

1. _____
2. _____
3. _____
4. _____
5. _____
6. _____
7. _____
8. _____
9. _____

ARENAVIRUSES

1. Rodents are the reservoir
2. No arthropod vector
3. Man gets infected by contact, inhalation of infectious animal excreta (LCM)
4. Man-to-man transmission also occurs (Lassa fever)

RUBELLA VIRUS

Properties

Enveloped virus, which contains single-stranded RNA, and replicates in the cytoplasm. There is only one serotype. The rubella virus is classified with Togaviruses; however, it is NOT an arthropod-borne disease, but rather is droplet spread

Clinical feature of postnatal rubella

1. There is enlargement of lymph nodes with conjunctivitis, often followed by a fine macular rash; slight fever may occur

2. The main risk of this infection is that it may occur in a non-immune woman during the first trimester of pregnancy, with serious consequences for the fetus

Clinical features of prenatal rubella

1. The risk of congenital malformations is greatest when the mother is infected during the first trimester of pregnancy
2. One or more of the following features may be present:
   a. Blindness
   b. Deafness
   c. Congenital heart defects
   d. Mental retardation (often with microcephaly)

Rubella virus is

1. DNA/RNA.

2. single/double stranded.

3. naked/enveloped.

4. multiplied in the nucleus/cytoplasm.

Replication of Rubella virus occurs in

the following stages (see Viral

Replication section)

1. _____

2. _____

3. _____

4. _____

194

RHABDOVIRUSES

Properties of the group
1. Bullet-shaped enveloped viruses, which contain single-stranded RNA, have a helical nucleocapsid, replicate in the cytoplasm, and are released by budding.
2. The group includes the virus responsible for rabies

Rabies

Serotypes: There is only one serotype of rabies virus

Epidemiology
1. The natural hosts include many kinds of mammals especially bats and skunks
2. The usual mode of transmission is by inoculation (bite). Infection may rarely result from inhalation of infective aerosols from bat secretions

Pathogenesis
1. Virus spreads along nerves to the CNS.
2. The virus causes destruction of nerve cells and demyelination; the highest concentration is usually found in the hippocampus

Artificially-acquired immunity

Vaccines
1. Virus is grown in human diploid cells and inactivated. Weekly, SubQ injections for 4 to 6 weeks are adequate. Human cell source virus has resulted in significant decrease in neurologic complications of vaccination
2. Passive antibody in the form of rabies immune globulin is also available

Treatment
1. Wound must be thoroughly cleansed
2. Inject rabies immune globulin (human origin) into the wound and I M
3. Start the vaccine immediately at another site

Diagnosis
1. Detain animal and observe for signs
2. Examine brain for Negri bodies

THE NEGRI BODY IS THE INCLUSION SEEN IN THE CYTOPLASM OF CELLS IN THE HIPPOCAMPUS AND OTHER CNS AREAS.

The replication cycle of the rabies virus

includes the following stages

(see Viral Replication section)

1 _____

2 _____

3. _____

4. _____

195

PICORNAVIRUSES

There are 2 groups of small (pico) RNA viruses, the enteroviruses and the rhinoviruses

ENTEROVIRUSES

Properties of the group

1. Naked viruses, icosahedral nucleocapsid, contain single-stranded RNA, and replicate in the cytoplasm

2. There are 4 subgroups: polioviruses, coxsackieviruses, echoviruses, and hepatitis A

Pathology
1. Most infections are subclinical

2. Virus multiplies first in the pharynx, small intestines and local lymph nodes

3. Viremia follows, with spread of virus to the brain and spinal cord

Polioviruses

1. A formalin-inactivated viral vaccine (Salk) containing all 3 serotypes is available for injection

2. A live attenuated viral vaccine (Sabin) containing either a single serotype or all 3 are given orally. It induces sIgA in addition to IgG and IgM and imparts immunity of long duration. May be dangerous in immunosuppressed individuals (use Salk vaccine)

3. Clinical diseases
    a. Most cases are subclinical
    b. Aseptic meningitis
    c. Poliomyelitis-an acute disease which causes flaccid paralysis. The virus replicates in many cells in the body. The target cells are the motor neurons in the CNS where destruction causes paralysis

There are 5 virus groups classified as small RNA viruses

1. _____

2. _____

3. _____

4. _____

5. _____

A. Salk vaccine

B. Sabin vaccine

C. Both

D. Neither

1. Confers intestinal immunity

2. Confers immunity to viremic phase of infection

3. Not recommended for patients with Bruton's disease

(answers on next page)

196

Coxsackieviruses

These viruses are classified as either A
or B depending on their pathogenicity for
mice

Clinical features

Infection may be inapparent, or result in
illness ranging in severity as far as
lethal disease. Several different forms
of illness can develop as follows:

1. Herpangina (vesicular pharyngitis) is
   the commonest manifestation of
   infection by A-serotypes
2. "Aseptic" meningitis can be caused by
   some A-serotypes or any B-serotypes
3. Epidemic myalgia is a common manifestation of infection by B-serotypes
4. Myocarditis or pericarditis can occur
   in infants from a B-serotype infection, and B-serotypes occasionally
   cause a myocardiopathy in children or
   adults

Echoviruses
Clinical features

1. Meningitis is commonly caused by
   echoviruses, but permanent paralysis is
   very rare
2. Skin rashes, pharyngitis and fever may
   occur
3. Echoviruses are a cause of a cold-like
   disease
4. Gastroenteritis and infantile diarrhea
   have been associated with echovirus
   infection

Hepatitis A is considered to be in this
group as well. (cf section on hepatitis
viruses for more information on this
agent)

answers
  1 = B
  2 = C
  3 = B
  4 = A
  5 = A, B
  6 = B
  7 = B

Match the disease with the Coxsackie

virus.

serotype A

serotype B

_____ 4. vesicular pharyngitis

_____ 5. aseptic meningitis

_____ 6. myocarditis

_____ 7. pericarditis

(answers at left, bottom)

Chemically pure
picornaviral RNA
CAN/CAN NOT
produce progeny
when introduced
into host cells.

197

RHINOVIRUSES

Properties of the group
Naked icosahedral viruses, contain single-stranded RNA

Serotypes:

More than 100 serotypes are known

1. These viruses are the commonest cause of the common cold (rhinitis, rhinorrea)
2. Rhinoviruses usually remain localized in the nasal mucosa

Artificially-acquired immunity

In view of the number of serotypes, the development of a vaccine is not practicable

CALICIVIRUSES

RNA virus which is single stranded. Etiologically associated with sporadic acute gastroenteritis in children

REOVIRUSES

Properties of the group
1. Naked icosahedral viruses, contain double-stranded RNA
2. Reoviruses can be isolated from feces and respiratory secretions of healthy persons, as well as from patients with a variety of illnesses, e.g., rhinitis
3. Rotaviruses cause gastroenteritis in human infants and lower animals
   a. most common cause of viral gastro-enteritis in the US; cause 70% of diarrheal disease seen by a US pediatrician.
   b. may cause 5-10% of adult diarrheas
   c. virus identified by ELISA

CORONAVIRUSES

Enveloped helical viruses, contain RNA; Coronaviruses are a common cause of a cold-like disease in adults, but they do not seem to be an important cause of acute respiratory illness in children

Match the disease with the virus

   A. Norwalk agent

   B. Reovirus

   C. Rhinovirus

   D. Rotovirus

1. Rhinitis

2. Gastroenteritis in adults

3. Gastroenteritis in infants

(answers at bottom)

Viruses with dsRNA include

1. _____

2. _____

Answers
   1. B, C
   2. A
   D. D

NORWALK AGENT

Cause of diarrheal disease in infants less than two years of age; disease occurs both in epidemics as well as sporodically

HEPATITIS VIRUSES

Viral hepatitis types A and B

Three particular forms of viral hepatitis can be distinguished clinically; these are hepatitis type A (infectious hepatitis or short- incubation hepatitis) = RNA virus; hepatitis type B (serum hepatitis or long-incubation hepatitis) = DNA virus and; non A-/non B hepatitis (disease resembles that of type B). There are multiple causes of non A-non B hepatitis including Hepatitis C and E; hepatitis A is now enterovirus 72

Incubation period

Type A: 10 to 50 days
Type B: 50 to 180 days
Non A, Non B: 50 to 180 days

Signs and symptoms

The illness is characterized by malaise, anorexia, nausea, vomiting, diarrhea, fever and also jaundice which may or may not appear between two days and three weeks after onset

Type A: In young children, infection frequently remains inapparent or develops into a mild illness without jaundice; in older age groups, infection often leads to icterus or more severe disease

Type B: The Dane particle is the infectious entity. Infection may remain inapparent. Many cases continue to chronic hepatitis with surface antigen carrier state. Primary hepatocellular carcinoma may develop

Type C: The leading cause of post-transfusion hepatitis. High incidence of chronic liver disease; cirrhosis and hepatocellular carcinoma common. Interferon α approved for therapy.

Type D: A defective virus that replicates only in Hepatitis B-infected cells.   Needs HBsAg for capsid. Delta antigen is unique. Uncommon in US; seen mainly in Italy and the Middle East.

Which of the following agents of viral hepatitis can be transmitted via transfusion?

1.   Hepatitis A

2.   Hepatitis B

3.   Hepatitis C

4.   Hepatitis D

5.   Hepatitis E

[answer at bottom of page]

Hepatitis D virus is

defective; it needs

_____ which

is/are supplied by

_____.

Serious, life threatening

complications of hepatitis

B and C viral diseases

include _____

and _____.

Therapy for chronic hepatitis

includes _____.

The incubation period for

Hepatitis B is _____.

[answer = all are possible]

Type E: Enterically transmitted calicivirus (naked ssRNA) disease seen mainly in Far East. Mortality rate of 20% in pregnant women.

Epidemiology

All may be transmitted via blood during viremic stage but HAV and HEV are also spread via fecal/oral route.

Laboratory diagnosis

Serum is examined in a "hepatitis profile" that looks for the following viral markers; anti-HAV IgM, HBsAg, anti-HB IgM and anti-HCV.

Therapy

Immune serum globulin useful for HAV, HBV and HCV exposures. Interferonα used for chronic hepatitis, especially HCV.

Prophylaxis

Vaccine available for HBV; either purified HBsAg from human plasma or recombinant vaccine using HBsAg gene.

The presence of HBsAg in

serum means _____

_____

_____

_____.

The two viral hepatitides

that are spread by the

Fecal/Oral route are

_____, and

_____.

_____ is

the cause of high mortality

in pregnant Asian women.

SIGNIFICANCE OF HEPATITIS B ANTIGENS AND ANTIBODIES IN SERUM

Component Present in Serum

HBsAg	Anti-HBs	Anti-HBc	Interpretation
+	−	−	Prodromal period or early acute disease. Person is considered infectious.
+	−	+	Acute disease or chronic carrier. Person is considered infectious.
−	+	+	Convalescing from the disease or immune.
−	+	−	Immune via disease or vaccination.
−	−	+	Recovered from disease and lost reactivity. Antibody of IgG class; low level. or Recent disease; serum taken after HBsAg disappeared, before anti-HBs. Anti-HBc should be high. Such people are infectious.

SLOW VIRUSES

Diseases caused by viruses and virus-like agents belonging to different taxonomic groups, and linked together by the fact that they are all characterized by spongiform encephalopathy, and a long incubation period. Some of these agents may be PRIONS, small proteinaceous infectious particles

Subacute sclerosing panencephalitis (SSPE)

Infectious measles virus has been isolated from brain tissue and lymph nodes of affected individuals with a history of measles

Kuru

The disease seems to have resulted from cannibalism. Kuru has been found only in a single tribe in New Guinea

Progressive Multifocal leukoencephalopathy

A rare disease of the CNS. Papovavirus JC has been isolated from affected tissues

Creutzfeldt-Jakob disease

A rare disease of the CNS which has been transmitted to chimpanzees by inoculation of material from the brains of patients

Multiple sclerosis

A CNS disease suspected to be of viral etiology. There is serological evidence suggesting that measles virus may be involved

Match the virus with the disease

    A. measles

    B. JC papovavirus

1. multiple sclerosis

2. subacute sclerosing panencephalitis

3. progressive multifocal leukoencephalopathy

(answers at bottom of page)

1=A
2=A
3=B

ONCOGENIC VIRUSES

Properties of oncogenic viruses

1. Among the RNA viruses, only <u>Retroviridae</u> are oncogenic
   a. the Oncornavirus group causes tumors in diverse animal species; HTLV-I and II are the human pathogens
   b. the Lentiviruses are in the same family: these are the slow viruses of spongiform encephalopathies; Human immunodeficiency virus is not oncogenic (does not contain an oncogene) but is associated with certain cancers
2. Oncogenic DNA viruses that cause tumors in humans are found in the Papova, Hepadna, and Herpesvirus families
3. It appears that some or all of the genes of some oncogenic viruses may be integrated into host DNA; the RNA viruses being integrated by an RNA-dependent DNA polymerase (reverse transcriptase). Integration is essential for oncogenesis.

Transformation in vitro

The properties of transformed cells include:

1. Loss of contact inhibition

2. Altered cell morphology

3. The presence of new antigens in the membrane (tumor specific transplantation antigens) and intracellularly

4. The ability to proliferate rapidly with concomitant high energy demand

5. Altered chromosomal morphology and/or number
6. Ability to grow in soft agar and produce tumors when injected into an appropriate host

HEPADNAVIRUS

Hepatitis B virus is associated with hepatocellular carcinoma in humans

Oncogenesis by DNA Viruses

Early proteins produced during viral infection have many functions, including **activation** of cellular biosynthetic processes and **down-regulation** of others. In viral oncogenesis some of these proteins **bind to cellular ANTI-oncogenes and inactivate their growth suppressing functions**, thus permitting uncontrolled proliferation of the infected cell. In most instances the viral replicative cycle is not completed, so that the cells do not have overt evidence of the viral infection. Thus following a viral infection the cell has two paths it might follow - productive infection with release of infectious virus, or transformation to malignancy.

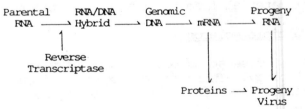

Replication of Retroviruses

Retroviral reverse transcriptase has four catalytic functions:
1. RNA-dependent DNA polymerase
2. DNA-dependent DNA polymerase
3. RNAse which degrades the RNA in the RNA-DNA hybrid
4. Integrase which inserts viral DNA into the host genome

POXVIRUSES

Molluscum contagiosum virus in this group cause benign skin lesions

HERPESVIRUSES

1. In lower animals these viruses cause Marek's disease (a neurolymhomatosis) in chickens, renal carcinoma in frogs and other malignancies
2. Epstein-Barr virus is associated with Burkitt's lymphoma in young African boys and nasopharyngeal carcinoma in certain ethnics groups in southern China. Consumption of cantonese-style salted fish during childhood appears to be a co-factor

PAPOVAVIRUSES

1. Papillomaviruses

   a. These cause benign papillomas (warts) in man and other mammalian species. In man, condyloma acuminatum causes genital wart which are usually benign
   b. Human papilloma virus # 16 causes cervical carcinoma

Polyomavirus

   It induces the formation of sarcomas and carcinomas in diverse animal species; not in humans

3. SV 40 virus and Adenoviruses

   In experimental conditions, they induce malignant neoplasms in mice, and causes transformation in vitro of cells of many species.

Human DNA viruses are associated with following cancers

1. _____

2. _____

3. _____

RETROVIRUSES

1. These enveloped viruses contain single-stranded RNA; the virion also contains reverse transcriptase which, together with certain other enzymes, produces double-stranded DNA homologous to the virion RNA. This goes to the nucleus and becomes integrated into the cellular DNA as a provirus which may be transcribed by a DNA-dependent RNA polymerase to make RNA copies, some of which are viral genome and some act as mRNA
2. The oncogene hypothesis proposes that the viral genome consists of at least 2 sets of genes, one of which controls the process of oncogenesis, and the other the production of infectious virus; either, neither or both sets may be evoked by endogenous or exogenous factors
3. Retroviruses can activate host genes (e.g., the c-myc gene)

SAMPLE RETROVIRUS GENOME

gag	pol	env

The gag gene encodes capsid proteins, which are synthesized as a polyprotein precursor and then split by a protease. The pol gene encodes reverse transcriptase. The env gene encodes glycoprotein spikes in the envelope. Additional genes in the env region include tat which encodes a transactivator that enhances expression of all viral genes, rev which is required for expression of gag, pol, and env, and nef which down regulates HIV genome replication.

VIRUSES AND HUMAN CANCER

Burkitt's lymphoma

Specific antigen and nucleic acid of
Epstein-Barr (EBNA) herpesvirus is
present in cells cultured from cases of
Burkitt's B cell lymphoma. This virus
also appears to be responsible for
infectious mononucleosis. Patients with
Burkitt's lymphoma have a high incidence
and high titers of antibody against EB
virus

Nasopharyngeal carcinoma

herpesvirus has been detected in cells
obtained from cases of nasopharyngeal
carcinoma, and patients show high titers
of anti-EB herpesvirus antibody

Carcinoma of the uterine cervix

Papilloma virus, serotype 16, seems to be
etiologically associated with cervical
cancer

Hepatocellular Carcinoma

Hepatitis B virus has been associated
with primary carcinoma of the liver

Kaposi's Sarcoma

1. Human Immunodeficiency Virus 1 (HIV),
    a Retrovirus, is etiologically
    associated with Kaposi's sarcoma and
    AIDS. It is antigenically different
    from all other retroviruses.
2. Individuals with AIDS suffer from
    infections by opportunists such as
    Pneumocystis, Candida, Cryptococcus
    and Cryptosporidium. CMV infections
    are often activated.
3. There will be inverted CD4:CD8
    lymphocyte ratios (due to the CD4
    "target" of this virus) and normal to
    elevated levels of IgG, etc. The
    disease is particularly common in
    homosexuals, hemophiliacs, and intra-
    venous drug users. Neonates are
    involved via transplacental passage
    of the virus. Heterosexual trans-
    mission is common in Africa.

The most common mechanism of viral
oncogenesis is insertional activation of the oncogene. In neoplastic
cells a new provirus is found in
close proximity to the c-myc proto-
oncogene. The provirus is usually
but always contains one LTR (long
terminal repeat) units which are very
important in integration of the viral
DNA into that of the cell and also
serve as an enhancer to activate
the c-myc gene and deregulate cell
proliferation.

GENETIC STRUCTURE OF THE RETROVIRUSES

FOUR MAIN GENES
  gag = codes for nucleocapsid proteins
  Pro = codes for protease
  Pol = codes for polymerase enzymes
        reverse transcriptase
        integrase
  Env = codes for envelope proteins

HUMAN T-CELL LYMPHOTROPIC VIRUSES

A human Retrovirus has been
isolated from numerous cases
of adult T-cell leukemia and
lymphoma. The HTLV agents
have a marked affinity for
mature T cells. Clusters of
HTLV disease have been
reported from the Caribbean
basin and the southern United
States.

REVIEW STATEMENTS

These should be used to strengthen and expand your understanding of Pathogenic Microbiology. If you are uncertain about the veracity of a statement, please "check it out." This will help you strengthen your grasp of the material. You may wish to develop your own list. If you have a spare sheet of paper available, write down the correct statement for every question you miss in going through review exams. This way you can avoid marking on the review exam (so you can use it again) and still have captured that fact for future review.

The **major virulence** factor of the **pneumococcus** is the **capsular carbohydrate**. It aids in the invasiveness of the agent by virtue of its antiphagocytic action. The vaccine is composed of capsular antigens from the 23 most common types.

Streptococcus pneumoniae produces alpha hemolysis on blood agar; the pneumococci are differentiated from the green (viridans) streptococci by their sensitivity to **optochin**.

The antibiotic of choice for pneumococcal pneumonia is **pencillin**.

Group A beta hemolytic streptococci are differentiated from other beta hemolytic streptoccci by their **sensitivity to bacitracin.**

Two **antiphagocytic** surface components of Group A streptococci are the **M protein** and **hyaluronic acid**; the latter is not antigenic.

Erythrogenic toxin is produced only by lysogenic strains of streptococci.

The extracellular product of streptococci which converts plasminogen to plasmin is **streptokinase** (fibrinolysin). It is used to treat heart attack victims.

Acute glomerulonephritis is associated with group A streptococcal infections of either skin or upper respiratory tract.

Staphylococci are **resistant to penicillin** by virtue of a plasmid-conferred enzyme, **beta lactamase**.

Staphylococcal carriers are identified in epidemiologic studies (e.g., hospital nurseries) by bacteriophage sensitivity patterns.

Surface components of the staphylococcus which are **anti-phagocytic** include **capsule** and **protein A**.

Streptococcus pneumoniae is the most a common cause of bacterial **pneumonia in adults**.

Aerobic Gram negative diplococci belong to the genus *Neisseria*.

N. meningitidis is divided into four **serologic types** on the basis of antigenic difference of the capsular carbohydrate; the **majority of meningococcal epidemics are caused by type A.**

The acute adrenal insufficiency seen in fulminating cases of meningococcemia is called the **Waterhouse-Friderichsen syndrome.**

The surface components of the **meningococcus** which are involved in its pathogenicity include the **capsule** and **endotoxin**. Pili are responsible for the organism's interaction with host cell membranes.

Pili are found on the virulent strains of **gonococci**, types I and II.

Gonorrhea may be an asymptomatic infection, particularly in females. Gonorrhea can be diagnosed in males (only) by the observation of **Gram negative diplococci inside PMN's.**

In addition to "a flow of seed" the gonococcus also causes **arthritis,** and **ophthalmia neonatorum.**

The treatment of choice for neisserial infections is **penicillin**; if dealing with a penicillinase producing strain of gonococci, **spectinomycin** or **ceftriaxone** should be used.

Primary atypical pneumonia (as a disease entity) may be caused by various chlamydial and viral agents; however, it is most closley associated with *Mycoplasma pneumoniae.*

Penicillins and cephalosporins are not indicated in the **treatment of mycoplasmal infections** because these are inhibitors of cell wall synthesis and mycoplasma do not have a cell wall. Diseases caused by mycoplasma can be treated with **tetracyclines**.

The most common serologic tests for the identification of *Mycoplasma pneumoniae* (although they rely on heterophile antigens) are cold hemagglutinins and Strep MG agglutinins.

The two genera of **Gram positive rods** which form spores are *Clostridium* and *Bacillus*; the former will only grow anaerobically.

The two major virulence factors of the **anthrax bacillus** are the **polypeptide capsule** and anthrax **toxin**. The anthrax toxin is somewhat unique in biology in that its lethal effect on the host is due to the synergistic action of 3 proteins.

Although **gas gangrene** can be caused by serveral clostridia, the species most commonly associated with this disease entity is *perfringens*.

Three toxic enzymes which are of particular importance in **gas gangrene** are **lecithinase, collagenase** and **hyaluronidase.**

A common feature in the **treatment of clostridial** infections is the use of specific **antitoxin**.

Gas gangrene and tetanus are both contracted via soil contamination of wounds; their clinical pictures differ markedly in that **gangrene is an invasive process** whereas **tetanus is** a very **localized** infection the symtoms of which are due to **toxemia**.

Botulism is an intoxication caused by an organism which elaborates a potent heat labile **neurotoxin** in which acts on the autonomic nervous system and **interferes with transmission of nerve impulses at the myoneural junction.**

The etiologic agent of **Hansen's disease** has not been grown *in vitro*. Leprosy is thought to be transmitted to man via direct contact or respiratory droplet. Leprosy can be diagnosed by skin testing with an extract of lepromatous nodules referred to as **lepromin.**

Diphtheria is most effectively treated by the administration of specific **antitoxin;** antibiotics are insufficient alone because most of the symptomatology is due to the organism's excretion of toxin.

Three classical enteric diseases are **typhoid, dysentery,** and **cholera,** caused by *Salmonella, Shigella,* and *Vibrio,* respectively.

The chemical composition of **endotoxin** is **lipopolysacchride; lipid A** is the **toxic** moiety.

Escherichia coli is the most common cause of **urinary tract infections**.

Capsular carbohydrate is a major virulence factor of *Klebsiella pneumoniae*.

Shigella dysenteriae produces an **A-B exotoxin** that is an enterotoxin in man.; it inhibits protein synthesis.

The pathogenesis of *Vibrio cholerae* is dependent upon **choleragen,** an **A-B enterotoxin** which increases **adenyl cyclase** activity. **Rice-water stools**, fluid and electrolyte loss, and eventual **hypovolemic shock** are characteristics of cholera.

Of all the enteric bacilli *Salmonella typhi* is the most likely to be **isolated from blood**.

An **antiphagocytic polysaccharide capsule** similar to that of *S. pneumoniae* is a virulence factor of *Haemophilus influenzae*.

The etiologic agent of **whooping cough** is *Bordetella pertussis*. Heat-killed organisms are employed in the DPT vaccine; the **acellular** vaccine contains **pertussis toxoid.**

Yersinia pestis may be transmitted by **rat fleas** and human lice.

Brucella abortus demonstrates **a tissue tropism** in cattle since the organisms localize in the **placenta** which contains a high concentration of erythritol. The virulence of *Brucella* is attributed to their ability to resist intracellular killing.

There are three genera of spirochetes that cause human disease; *Leptospira, Treponema* and *Borrelia*. Two genera are **zoonotic** in nature (i.e., infect animals primarily with man as an incidental host); *Leptospira* and *Borrelia*. The primary organs affected in **leptospirosis** are the **liver** and **kidneys**. The agents causing the other spirochetal diseases are more diverse in their distribution throughout the body. **Leptospirosis** is contracted via **exposure to contaminated water**; **Lyme disease** occurs after **tick (Ixodes) bites**.

Scarlet fever is a local infection with toxemia (**erythrogenic toxin**).

Chlamydia trachomatis is the most common cause of sexually transmitted disease in the United States.

A rise in **antistreptolysin-O titer** or anti DNAse B is an indication of recent infection with *Streptococcus pyogenes*.

Man is the only natural host for *Neisseria meningitidis*. Persons with meningococcal pharyngitis may fail to develop meningitis. Meningococcal petechial hemorrhages often contain *Neisseria meningitidis*.

In the routine **diagnosis of diphtheria**, positive identification of *Corynebacterium diphtheriae* is made by demonstration of its ability to **produce diphtheria toxin**.

BCG, which is used for active immunization against tuberculosis, consists of **attentuated bovine tubercle bacilli.**

The production of a water soluble, **blue-green pigment** in a culture indicates the presence of *Pseudomonas aeruginosa*.

The spirochetes associated with fusospirochetal infections, as well as the etiologic agents of relapsing fever, belong to **the genus *Borrelia*;** Lyme disease is caused by *B. burgdorferi*.

Malarial relapses are due primarily to emergence of persisting **exoerythrocytic merozoites.**

Fatal malaria most often results from infection with *Plasmodium falciparum*.

Haemophilus influenzae causes life-threatening **epiglottitis in neonates.**

One virulence factor of *Mycobacterium tuberculosis* is the **cord factor** (6, 6' trehalose dimycolate).

During oral antibiotic therapy (e.g., **clindamycin**), a patient may develop **pseudomembranous enterocolitis** caused by *Clostridium difficile.*

Enterobius is the most common helminth parasite infection of children in the United States. Enterobius female worms lay their eggs on the perianal skin and cause **pruritis.** Anal impression smears can be made to detect these eggs. **Pinworm** is treated with **mebendazole.**

The potential for **autoinfection** makes *Strongyloides* a dangerous infection, especially in the **immunologically compromised host.**

Myalgia, **ocular edema** and **eosinophilia** are symptoms associated with symptomatic **trichinosis.**

Adult **tapeworm infections** are acquired by ingesting animal tissue that harbors the larvae stage, e.g., *Taenia solium* in pork and *T. saginata* in beef. Cysticerosis may occur if man ingests *Taenia solium* eggs.

Diphyllobothrium latum competes with the host for Vitamin B_{12}, this competition occasionally results in **pernicious anemia.**

Entamoeba histolytica may cause **abscesses** in the large bowel with secondary lesions in other organs, especially the **liver.**

Giardiasis is the most common protozoan diarrheal infection of man in the United States. Symptoms include **flatulence, foul smelling stools**, nausea and cramping; the disease is common in **day care centers.**

Numerous pathogens secrete an **IgA protease** which aids in infectivity; e.g., *H. influenzae, Neisseria gonorrhoeae, N. meningitidis, Streptococcus pneumoniae, mitis*, and *sanguis*, and *Bacteroides spp.*

Candida albicans is a part of the **normal flora**.

Fungi are **resistant** to most **antibacterial** chemotherapeutic **agents**.

Clinical malaria is best treated with **chloroquine**. **Primaquine** is necessary to eradicate persisting exoerythrocytic liver stages of *Plasmodium vivax*.

Metronidazole is an effective drug for treating *Trichomonas vaginalis*. Sexual partner(s) must also be treated to prevent reinfection.

Bacteroides are the predominant **flora of the gut;** they are anaerobic gram negative rods.

Actinomycosis is characterized by 1) an **endogenous origin** of the anaerobic infectious agent,and 2) **sulfur granules** in exudate of lesion which are really masses of Gram positive rods.

Cryptococcus neoformans is the **ONLY encapsulated yeast** that is pathogenic for man. It is identified by India ink preparations of spinial fluid.

Schistosomiasis is acquired by **larval penetration of the skin**; the larvae develop in snail hosts in fecally contaminated waters.

The etiologic agent of human **warts** (verrucae) is a **papovavirus.**

Commercially available **influenza vaccine** contains inactivated influenza viruses, **types A and B.**

Coxsackie A and B viruses cause **herpangina** and **myocarditis**, respectively. Coxsackie viruses of Group B are responsible for a considerable proportion of cases of aseptic meningitis.

The **hepatitis B surface antigen** (HBsAg), when found in banked blood, renders it undesirable for use in blood transfusions. The **incubation period** of serum hepatitis usually ranges from **50-180 days.**

The finding of **Negri bodies** (cytoplasmic inclusions in neurons) is specific for the pathologic diagnosis of **rabies.**

Rhinoviruses are acid labile and hence can not survive the acidity of the stomach; they do not colonize the GI tract as do the other Picornaviruses.

Measles is prevented by administration of an attenuated **monovalent vaccine**. It may be included with rubella and mumps vaccines to produce a polyvalent product.

Clinical signs and symptoms of **measles** include **photophobia**, cough, coryza, conjunctivitis and **Koplik spots.** Complications of measles include **encephalitis** and **pneumonia. Subacute sclerosing panencephalitis** is thought to be caused by measles.

Mumps is a disease of secretory cells which may involve the pancreas. Following the initial attack of mumps, long lasting protective immunity is produced. Mumps is spread from the infected patient by droplets (aerosol) or fresh fomites.

Type A influenza viruses are known to cause **pandemics** while types B and C influenza viruses are less likely to do so. Antibodies to the hemagglutinin spikes of influenza viruses are protective.

Antigenic drift is brought about by minor changes in type A influenza viruses while **antigenic shift** involves major changes in one or more of the glycoprotein spikes.

Translocation of the c-myc gene to one of the immunoglobulin gene loci is characteristic of **Burkitt's lymphoma,** but is not seen in infectious mononucleosis.

Parainfluenza viruses cause bronchitis, **bronchiolitis** and **croup** in children and a common cold-like disease in adults. **Respiratory syncytial virus** commonly produces severe disease (bronchitis, bronchiolitis and pneumonia) in infants.

The portal of entry of **enteroviruses** is the oral cavity and the viruses invade through the oropharyngeal and intestinal mucosa. They spread throughout the body via the lymphatics and blood. **Polio vaccines** must be polyvalent as there are **3 antigenically distinct viruses.** The **Sabin** polio vaccine contains **attenuated** virus which is taken **orally** while the Salk polio vaccine is formalin-inactivated and is administered by injection.

Coxsackie B viruses are responsible for many cases of **aseptic meningitis.**

Rhabdoviruses are single stranded, RNA-containing, bullet shaped viruses; **Rabies** virus is a rhabdovirus. Rabies virus is usually spread by the bite or lick of a rabid animal. The rabies vaccine of choice contains **inactive human diploid cell** produced virus.

Type A hepatitis is spread primarily by the **fecal-oral** route and **type B hepatitis** is spread primarily by **injection** but both viruses can be spread by either route. **Hepatitis C** is spread primarily by **injection.** **Hepatitis E** is spread by fecal-oral route

Rotaviruses are REO viruses which are the causal agents of **infantile diarrhea**, a particularly severe disease in the very young.

Pharyngeal-conjunctival fever is the most common syndrome associated with **adenoviruses.**

Kuru (a disease seen in New Guinea) and **Creutzfeldt-Jacob diseases** are transmissable **spongiform encephalopathies** of humans.

Rubella virus belongs to the **Togavirus** family. Lasting protective immunity is usually produced upon convalescence from rubella. Rubella virus is known to **cross the human placenta** and to infect the developing fetus. **Congenital rubella** is the result of fetal infection during the **first trimester** of pregnancy. Following birth, virus may be excreted and cause a rubella outbreak in a newborn nursery. An **attenuated viral vaccine** is effective in the prevention of rubella but should not be given to pregnant humans.

The **Epstein-Barr virus** (EBV) has been recovered from **Burkitt's lymhoma** tissue, from human patients with **nasopharyngeal carcinomas,** and from patients with **infectious mononucleosis.**

Reactivation of a latent infection in the form of **shingles** (Herpes zoster) occurs with the etiologic agent of varicella (chicken pox). **Zoster** (shingles) is a recurrent disease; the lesions appear unilaterally on the body, in a **dermatome** distribution.

Herpes simplex virus may cause **cold sores** and **aseptic meningitis.** Herpes simplex virus, type 2, is associated with genital herpes (lesions of genital tract) and neonatal herpes. **Acyclovir** has been used quite effectively in treating herpesvirus infections, including serious systemic infections.

Aspirin therapy in children with influenza or chickenpox is contraindicated due to the possible association of these conditions with **Reye syndrome.**

The predominant **cell in the spinal fluid** in **viral meningitis** is the **lymphocyte.** This is the same cell that would predominate in the **perivascular cuffing** also noted in these diseases.

Rotavirus is the most common cause of **pediatric infectious diarrhea** in the USA. *Campylobacter* spp. is the most common bacterial agent.

Adenoviruses are the most common cause of **viral pharyngitis;** among the bacteria, *Streptococcus pyogenes* is the most common, and is probably the most serious in light of the sequelae which can develop.

Retroviral RNA is transcribed into circular dsDNA and **inserted into the host genome** as an early event that precedes viral replication. Viral progeny and viral mRNA are made by transcription from this DNA.

Parainfluenza and **influenza viruses** are the most common cause of infections of the **larynx** and **bronchi;** viruses rarely affect the epiglottitis, however *Haemophilus influenzae* is a pathogen here.

PATHOGENIC MICROBIOLOGY REVIEW EXAM

SELECT THE SINGLE BEST COMPLETION FOR EACH QUESTION.

1. The virulence of *S. pneumoniae* is primarily associated with the presence of

   A. cell wall teichoic acid.
   B. pneumolysin.
   C. polysaccharide capsule.
   D. M protein.
   E. peptidoglycan.

2. Viruses for which there are effective, live vaccines include

   A. influenza A and coronavirus.
   B. mumps, rubella, and parvovirus.
   C. measles, mumps, and influenza A.
   D. rubella and measles.

3. Which of the following streptococcal diseases is caused in part by erythrogenic toxin?

   A. Impetigo
   B. Puerperal sepsis
   C. Rheumatic fever
   D. Scarlet fever
   E. Erysipelas

4. Which of the following would most likely be etiologically involved in meningitis in a 3 week old infant ?

   A. *Neisseria meningitidis*
   B. *Haemophilus influenzae*
   C. *Streptococcus pneumoniae*
   D. *Streptococcus agalactiae*
   E. *Listeria monocytogenes*

5. Vaccine induced immunity to pnemococcal pneumonia is of what type?

   A. Antitoxic
   B. Bacteriocidal
   C. Opsonic
   D. Bacteriolytic
   E. Neutralizing

6. Individuals vaccinated with the HB_SAg vaccine would be protected from infection by

   A. hepatitis A virus only.
   B. hepatitis B virus only.
   C. hepatitis C virus only.
   D. delta hepatitis virus only.
   E. Both hepatitis B and delta viruses.

7. What clinical condition may be produced by the germination of spores of *Clostridium botulinum* in the gastrointestinal tract of infants?

   A. Pseudomembranous enterocolitis
   B. Enteritis necroticans
   C. Lockjaw
   D. Floppy baby syndrome
   E. Rice water stools

8. A key characteristic of the etiologic agent of bacillary dysentery is

   A. strict localization of the pathogen in the small intestine.
   B. the organism is found mainly in animals.
   C. production of a potent cytotoxin responsible for invasiveness.
   D. the organism is transmitted by droplet aerosol.

9. What is the most common source of salmonellosis in the United States?

   A. Pet turtles
   B. Rare roast beef
   C. Potato salad
   D. Poultry products
   E. Partially cooked seafood

10. *Salmonella typhi* differs from other species of *Salmonella* in that it

    A. produces enteritis localized in the small intestine.
    B. is found mainly in animals.
    C. has a predilection for lymphoid tissues in the liver and spleen.
    D. produces a heat-stable enterotoxin.
    E. causes acute dysentery.

11. Which of the following are surface components of *Staphylococcus aureus* serves as an adherence molecule?

    A. Protein A
    B. Carbohydrate capsule
    C. Coagulase
    D. Teichoic acid
    E. Peptidoglycan

12. *Pseudomonas aeruginosa* strains isolated from cystic fibrosis patients are unique in that they

    A. are Gram positive.
    B. are obligate anaerobes.
    C. contain no endotoxin in the cell wall.
    D. produce mucoid colonies due to excess extracellular polysaccharide.
    E. produce an enterotoxin.

13. Which of the following vaccines could most safely be given to an immunosuppressed individual?

    A. Heptavax
    B. Sabin
    C. Yellow fever
    D. Rubella
    E. Mumps

14. The most common species of *Mycobacterium* isolated from AIDS patients is

    A. *Mycobacterium kansasii.*
    B. *Mycobacterium avium-intracellulare* complex.
    C. *Mycobacterium leprae.*
    D. *Mycobacterium phlei.*
    E. *Mycobacterium scrofulaceum.*

15. A diagnostic test that is used for the confirmation of infection with HIV is

    A. radioimmune assay (RIA).
    B. enzyme-linked immunosorbent assay (ELISA).
    C. Ouchterlony.
    D. Western blot assay.
    E. latex agglutination assay.

16. Mycobacteria resist intracellular killing due to which cell wall constituent?

    A. Lipopolysaccharide
    B. Lipoteichoic acid
    C. Periplasm
    D. Mycolic acids (wax D)
    E. Peptidoglycan

17. Blood and leukocytes are seen frequently in the stool during

    A. cholera.
    B. rotaviral diarrhea.
    C. shigellosis.
    D. salmonellosis.
    E. traveler's diarrhea.

18. In cryptococcal meningitis, the level of this substance in spinal fluid can be diagnostic as well as prognostic.

    A. Anticryptococcal IgM antibody
    B. Cryptococcal capsular carbohydrate
    C. CEA
    D. Anticryptococcal IgG antibody

19. Increasing levels of anti-Histoplasma complement-fixing antibody in the serum of a patient with histoplasmosis being treated with Amphotericin B is

    A. indicative of a poor prognosis.
    B. indicative of a good prognosis.
    C. of no prognostic value.
    D. a signal to stop treatment.

20. The cellular oncogene that is translocated from chromosome 8 to chromosome 14 in the majority of the cases of Burkitt's lymphoma is the

A. c-SRC gene.
B. c-MYC gene.
C. c-ERB gene.
D. c-RAS gene.

21. The antifungal activity of the polyene antibiotic Amphotericin B is related to its

A. accumulation in keratinized tissue.
B. intercalation in mitochondrial DNA.
C. interaction with membrane sterols.
D. inhibiting cross linking in fungal cell walls.
E. inhibition of DNA dependent RNA polymerase.

22. Which of the following fungal agents is an endogenous cause of human disease?

A. *Cryptococcus neoformans*
B. *Candida albicans*
C. *Trichophyton rubrum*
D. *Sporothrix schenckii*
E. *Histoplasma capsulatum*

23. In AIDS patients autoinfection is a possible consequence of infection with

A. Hookworm.
B. *Ascaris.*
C. *Strongyloides.*
D. *Trichuris.*

24. The extra-intestinal site most frequently affected in amebiasis is

A. lung.
B. liver.
C. genitalia.
D. brain.
E. skin.

25. Infectious hepatitis A

A. is frequently asymptomatic.
B. can be caused by different serotypes of HAV.
C. can only be transmitted by fecal-oral route.
D. often leads to a chronic state.

26. Which of the following properties would allow the physician to distinguish between HBV and HAV infections?

A. Jaundice
B. Fever
C. Alanine amino-transaminase (ALT) level
D. Incubation period

27. The most likely causative agent of amebic meningoencephalitis is

A. *Entamoeba histolytica.*
B. *Acanthoamoeba* sp.
C. *Entamoeba gingivalis.*
D. *Naegleria fowleri.*
E. *Giardia lamblia.*

28. The three genes contained by the majority of retroviruses are

A. gag, pol, tax
B. gag, onc, env
C. gag, pol, env
D. gag, env, env

29. The mode of transmission for *Schistosoma* is

A. fecal contamination (ingestion of eggs or cyst stage).
B. ingestion of fish.
C. larva penetrates skin.
D. ingestion of pork.
E. ingestion of beef.

30. The chemotherapeutic agent most appropriate for *Trichomonas* infection is

   A. metronidazole.
   B. avermectin.
   C. mebendazole.
   D. praziquantel.
   E. trimethoprim and sulfamethoxazole.

31. The major adherence factor of *Neisseria gonorrhoeae* is the

   A. lipopolysaccharide.
   B. pilus.
   C. capsule.
   D. M protein.
   E. teichoic acid.

32. Immunity to meningococcal infections is related to opsonizing and bactericidal antibodies to

   A. group specific polysaccharide (capsule).
   B. type specific M protein.
   C. pili variants.
   D. endotoxin.
   E. IgA protease.

33. Lyme disease is caused by *Borrelia burgdorferi*; the third stage of this disease is marked by the onset of

   A. arthritis.
   B. carditis.
   C. erythema chronicum migrans.
   D. peripheral neuropathy.
   E. atrioventricular heart block.

34. The most prevalent cause of sexually transmitted disease in the U.S. is

   A. Herpes virus.
   B. *Chlamydia trachomatis*.
   C. *Mycoplasma hominis*.
   D. *Neisseria gonorrhoeae*.
   E. *Treponema pallidum*.

35. What organism produces a frequently misdiagnosed food poisoning associated with fried rice?

   A. *Bacillus cereus*
   B. *Clostridium bifermentans*
   C. *Bacillus stearothermophilus*
   D. *Bacillus subtilis*
   E. *Clostridium perfringens*

36. The most serious sequela following infection of the genital mucous membranes in women with *Neisseria gonorrhoeae* or *Chlamydia trachomatis* is

   A. conjunctivitis.
   B. urethritis.
   C. pelvic inflammatory disease.
   D. salpingitis.
   E. proctitis.

37. ST toxin of *E. coli* is so called because it

   A. is heat stable.
   B. resembles shigella toxin.
   C. causes severe temperature rises.
   D. is also produced by *S. typhi*.
   E. causes shaking tremors.

38. The most appropriate treatment for systemic candidiasis is

   A. flucytosine.
   B. tolnaftate.
   C. ketoconazole.
   D. griseofulvin.
   E. nystatin.

39. The most common cause of urinary tract infection is

   A. *E. coli*.
   B. *S. aureus*.
   C. *K. pneumoniae*.
   D. *S. pyogenes*.
   E. *P. aeruginosa*.

40. Which of the following organisms has a cell wall with mycolic acids in it?

   A. *P. aeruginosa*
   B. *M. tuberculosis*
   C. *L. monocytogenes*
   D. *S. marcescens*
   E. *A. fumigatus*

41. A violent windstorm occurred in the San Joaquin Valley in California; the incidence of coccidioidomycosis increased sharply. This was due to spread of highly resistant

   A. spherules.
   B. arthroconidia.
   C. budding yeast.
   D. tuberculate chlamydospores.

42. A nineteen year old female was donating blood at her school blood drive. Routine screening revealed an elevated SGPT and the presence of Hepatitis B surface antigen. Which of the following is **FALSE?**

   A. Close contacts of this patient should receive Hepatitis B immune globulin.
   B. This patient has acute Hepatitis B infection.
   C. Prognosis cannot be determined at this time.
   D. Immediate liver biopsy is indicated.
   E. This patient is at risk of developing liver cancer.

43. Spore formation is important in the epidemiology of food poisoning caused by all of the following agents **EXCEPT**

   A. *Staphylococcus aureus.*
   B. *Bacillus cereus.*
   C. *Clostridium botulinum.*
   D. *Clostridium perfringens.*

44. It has been proposed that oncogenic retroviruses can transform cells to an oncogenic state by all of the following mechanisms **EXCEPT**

   A. Insertional mutagenesis
   B. Expression of oncogene present in virus
   C. Expression of tax gene
   D. Expression of vif gene

45. The enterotoxin of *Vibrio cholerae* does all of the following **EXCEPT**

   A. is composed of 1 A-subunit and 5 B-subunits.
   B. ADP-ribosylates the catalytic subunit of adenylate cyclase.
   C. localizes in the upper intestinal tract.
   D. increases intracellular cyclic-AMP.

46. Which of the following is **LEAST** likely to cause vaginitis?

   A. *Trichomonas vaginalis*
   B. *Candida albicans*
   C. *Treponema pallidum*
   D. *Gardnerella vaginalis*

47. All of the following are true about hepatitis C virus **EXCEPT**

   A. may cause chronic liver damage.
   B. is the primary cause of transfusion associated hepatitis.
   C. is an RNA virus.
   D. contain an envelope.
   E. it is defective

48. What characteristic listed below is **NOT** typical of *Clostridia?*

   A. Gram positive bacilli
   B. Facultative anaerobes
   C. Toxigenic
   D. Opportunistic pathogens
   E. Sporogenous

49. All of the following are associated with the cytomegalovirus **EXCEPT**

   A. congenital disease.
   B. heterophile antibody.
   C. latency.
   D. inclusion bodies.
   E. subclinical infections.

50. All of the following are characteristics of HIV **EXCEPT**

   A. contains it own oncogene.
   B. infects and damages cells of the CNS.
   C. contains several complex genes, including tat.
   D. is a member of the *Retroviridae* family.

214

51. All of the following would be likely members of the normal bacterial flora of the oral cavity **EXCEPT**

   A. *Staphylococcus aureus.*
   B. *Streptococcus pyogenes.*
   C. *Streptococcus salivarius.*
   D. *Neisseria pharyngis.*
   E. *Streptococcus mutans.*

52. Which of the following is **NOT** a pathway by which microbial toxins act?

   A. ADP ribosylation of host cell enzymes or control proteins.
   B. Activation of adenyl cyclase.
   C. Enhance neurotransmitter release from inhibitory neurons.
   D. Activation of guanyl cyclase.
   E. Activation of the complement cascade.

53. All of the following are chracteristics of endotoxin **EXCEPT**

   A. toxicity due to lipid A.
   B. heat stable.
   C. part of outer membrane of cell wall of Gram-negative bacteia.
   D. excellent immunogen.
   E. pyrogenic.

54. Etiologic agents of food poisoning include all of the following **EXCEPT**

   A. *Clostridum perfringens*
   B. *Bacillus cereus*
   C. *Salmonella typhimurium*
   D. *Salmonella typhi*
   E. *Escherichia coli*

55. Factors that appear to be important in the virulence of *Bordetella pertussis* include all of the following **EXCEPT**

   A. pertussis toxin
   B. pili
   C. capsule
   D. endotoxin
   E. IgA protease

56. Factors responsible for the pathogenicity of *Escherichia coli* include all of the following **EXCEPT**

   A. heat-labile enterotoxin.
   B. capsular (K) antigens.
   C. lipoteichoic acid adhesins.
   D. heat stable enterotoxin.
   E. endotoxin.

57. Epstein-Barr virus is associated with all of the following conditions **EXCEPT**

   A. Nasopharyngeal carcinoma
   B. Infectious mononucleosis
   C. Burkitt's lymphoma
   D. Systemic lupus erythematosus

58. Which of the following is **LEAST** likely in a mother who has a primary infection of rubella virus during pregnancy? The fetus may

   A. fail to develop signs of infections.
   B. be clinically normal but shed virus and have an IgM response.
   C. have virus-host cell interactions manifested by thrombocytopenia, hepatitis, or pneumonia.
   D. have virus-cell interactions manifested by heart malformation, cataracts, or mental retardation.
   E. handle the virus well and develop IgG antibodies.

59. Poliovirus vaccine is correctly described by all of the following statements **EXCEPT**

   A. The Sabin vaccine is a live attenuated virus cell-culture preparation.
   B. The Salk vaccine contains formalin-inactivated cell-culture prepared virus.
   C. It is a polyvalent preparation.
   D. Active virus is excreted in the feces of Sabin-vaccine-immunized individuals.
   E. The Sabin vaccine does not cause disease in humans.

MATCH THE INFECTIOUS AGENT WITH THE PATIENT DESCRIBED BELOW

A.	*Streptococcus pneumoniae*	G.	*Pseudomonas aeruginosa*
B.	*Klebsiella pneumoniae*	H.	*Viridans streptococci*
C.	*Mycoplasma pneumoniae*	I.	*Neisseria gonorrhoeae*
D.	*Streptococcus pyogenes*	J.	*Streptococcus mutans*
E.	*Legionella pneumophila*	K.	*Cryptococcus neoformans*
F.	*Staphylococcus aureus*	L.	*Serratia marcescens*

60.   This 16 year old white girl from Salt Lake City has a history of repeated streptococcal infections (pharyngitis) and cardiac abnormalities consistent with Rheumatic fever. Three weeks following extraction of an abscessed molar she develops fever and flu-like symptoms. Her condition worsens, a petechial rash appears, and she is hospitalized with a tentative diagnosis of subacute bacterial endocarditis caused by

61.   Lower respiratory tract infection associated with 1) a non-productive cough and lobar pneumonia, 2) mucoid sputum containing a paucity of bacteria upon Gram stain, 3) high serum titers of cold agglutinins, and 4) growth of "fried egg" colonies from the sputum on special laboratory agar indicates presumptive infection by

62.   A 4 year old child with a history of recurrent pulmonary infections has been brought to the Emergency room in obvious respiratory distress. Gram stain of the sputum reveals numerous polymorphonuclear neutrophils and gram positive cocci in grape-like clusters. The drug of choice to be employed until the antibiotic sensitivity report is received from the laboratory is methicillin. The agent most likely is

63.   A 32 year old female astronaut developed otitis media during a voyage in outer space. Culture yielded a gram positive coccus in chains which grew on blood agar with alpha hemolysis. The organism was catalase negative; growth was inhibited by optochin. The isolated organism can be identified as

64.   This 18 year old white male suffers from recurrent pulmonary problems associated with the cystic fibrosis disease which has plagued him all his life. He currently has pneumonia; the sputum stain reveals numerous Gram negative rods and PMNs. Cultures yield mixed flora with predominating mucoid colonies of a Gram negative bacillus. Antibiotic sensitivity tests are done on an isolate; the organism is found to be resistant to all antibiotics employed on the first plate. A green pigment is noted throughout the agar. The most likely organism is

65.   A 62 year old Caucasian housewife was admitted to the hospital complaining of intermittent frontal headaches, malaise, and vertigo. This woman was a diabetic and had been on corticosteroid therapy for approximately 6 months. The nurses noted that the patient was disoriented at times.
The patient's blood pressure was normal; temperature was 100°F. Skin tests with PPD, histoplasmin, and coccidioidin were negative. Chest X-ray showed nothing of significance.
Cerebrospinal fluid was obtained and the cell count showed 220 cells per cubic millimeter; they were predominantly lymphocytes. Total protein was slightly elevated; sugar was slightly decreased. Encapsulated yeast cells were observed in the sediment after centrifugation of the spinal fluid.

Disease

66. Pneumonia in AIDS patient

67. Post-neurosurgical meningitis

68. Localized skin infection in burn patient

Opportunist

A. *Aspergillus fumigatus*
B. *Pseudomonas aeruginosa*
C. *Staphylococcus epidermidis*
D. *Streptococcus salivarius*
E. *Pneumocystis carinii*
F. *Candida albicans*
G. *Streptococcus pneumoniae*
H. *Neisseria meningitidis*

Neoplasm

69. Kaposi's sarcoma

70. Primary liver carcinoma

71. Nasopharyngeal carcinoma

72. Burkitt's lymphoma

73. Cervical carcinoma

Virus

A. Hepatitis A virus
B. Hepatitis B virus
C. Hepatitis C virus
D. Hepatitis D virus
E. Herpes Simplex
F. Molluscum contagiosum
G. Papilloma virus
H. Parvovirus
I. Epstein Barr virus
J. Human immunodeficiency virus

Virus

74. Human immunodeficiency virus

75. Influenza A

76. Cytomegalovirus

77. Respiratory syncytial virus

78. Epstein Barr virus

79. Herpes zoster

80. Hepatitis C

Therapeutic agent

A. Amantadine
B. Acyclovir
C. Cytoxan
D. Adenine arabinoside
E. Pentamidine
F. Azidothymidine
G. Ganciclovir
H. Cyclosporin A
I. Ribavirin
J. Actinomycin D
K. Alpha interferon
L. Interleukin 2
M. Methisazone
N. Niclosamide

KEY

1.	C	21.	C	41.	B	61.	C
2.	D	22.	B	42.	D	62.	F
3.	D	23.	C	43.	A	63.	A
4	D	24.	B	44.	D	64.	G
5.	C	25.	A	45.	B	65.	K
6.	E	26.	D	46.	C	66.	E
7.	D	27.	D	47.	E	67.	C
8.	C	28.	C	48.	B	68.	B
9.	D	29.	C	49.	B	69.	J
10.	C	30.	A	50.	A	70.	B,C
11.	D	31.	B	51.	B	71.	I
12.	D	32.	A	52.	E	72.	I
13.	A	33.	A	53.	D	73.	G
14.	B	34.	B	54.	D	74.	F
15.	D	35.	A	55.	E	75.	A
16.	D	36.	C	56.	C	76.	G
17.	C	37.	A	57.	D	77.	I
18.	B	38.	A	58.	E	78.	B
19.	A	39.	A	59.	E	79.	B
20.	B	40.	B	60.	H	80.	K

COMPREHENSIVE REVIEW EXAMINATION

SELECT THE SINGLE BEST COMPLETION FOR EACH QUESTION BELOW.

1. The most common infection caused by *Salmonella* in the United States is

    A. gastroenteritis.
    B. septicemia.
    C. typhoid fever.
    D. paratyphoid fever.

2. The drug of choice for cryptococcosis is

    A. griseofulvin.
    B. amphotericin B.
    C. potassium iodide.
    D. nystatin.

3. The drug of choice for dermal, oral and vaginal candidiasis is

    A. griseofulvin.
    B. amphotericin B.
    C. potassium iodide.
    D. nystatin.

4. Sources of infection of Toxoplasma for humans include feces from

    A. cats.
    B. humans.
    C. dogs.
    D. dog fleas.
    E. dog ticks.

5. Infection of a susceptible cell with a hybrid virus which contains the genome of hepatitis A virus packaged inside the coat and envelope of an influenza virus would result in the production of

    A. hybrid virus with an influenza genome and a hepatitis A coat.
    B. influenza virus.
    C. hepatitis A virus.
    D. hybrid virus with a hepatitis genome and an influenza envelop.

6. The most common etiology of bacterial meningitis in the newborn is

    A. *Staphylococcus aureus.*
    B. *Streptococcus agalactiae*
    C. *Streptococcus pyogenes.*
    D. *Neisseria meningitidis.*
    E. *Haemophilus influenzae.*

7. The most common etiology of uncomplicated urinary tract infections is

    A. *Staphylococcus aureus.*
    B. *Escherichia coli.*
    C. *Streptococcus pyogenes.*
    D. *Neisseria meningitidis.*
    E. *Haemophilus influenzae.*

8. Neutrophil membrane constituents which aid in phagocytosis include receptors for

    A. C3b.
    B. Phytohemagglutinin.
    C. Fab.
    D. LPS.
    E. Clq.

9. A structure which contains lipid A, core polysaccharide and O-antigen would occur in an organism

    A. with ribitol teichoic acid in its cell wall.
    B. which is Gram negative.
    C. which forms spores.
    D. with adherence pili in its cell membrane.

10. The type of gene transfer that moves DNA from a donor cell to a recipient via a bacteriophage is

    A. transformation.
    B. transduction.
    C. conjugation.
    D. transacetylation.
    E. repression.

11. Hepatitis A virus

    A. is a helper virus for hepatitis delta agent.
    B. is transmitted primarily by the fecal-oral route.
    C. induces a chronic carrier state.
    D. causes hepatomas in a large number of cases.

219

12. The predominate cell in the spinal fluid of a child with aseptic meningitis is a (an)

   A. neutrophil.
   B. basophil.
   C. monocyte.
   D. eosinophil.
   E. lymphocyte.

13. A gram negative diplococcus was isolated from the cerebrospinal fluid of a twelve-year-old boy with acute purulent meningitis. It was oxidase positive and fermented glucose and maltose but not lactose. The organism most likely was

   A. *Neisseria meningitidis.*
   B. *Staphylococcus epidermidis.*
   C. *Escherichia coli.*
   D. *Staphylococcus aureus.*

14. The B portion of diphtheria toxin

   A. attaches to the membrane of susceptible cells.
   B. interferes with protein synthesis by inactivating elongation factor II.
   C. attaches to the 30S ribosome.
   D. attaches to the 50S ribosome.
   E. hydrolyzes NAD.

15. Increased levels of antibodies to Streptolysin O and DNAse in a patient's serum is indicative of a previous infection by

   A. *Neisseria gonorrhoeae.*
   B *Streptococcus mutans.*
   C. *Streptococcus pneumoniae.*
   D. *Streptococcus pyogenes.*
   E. *Staphylococcus aureus.*

16. A 4 year old child with a history of recurrent pulmonary infections has been brought to the emergency room in obvious respiratory distress. Numerous PMNs and gram positive coccus in grape like clusters were seen in the sputum. The drug of choice is

   A. penicillin.
   B. methicillin.
   C. streptomycin.
   D. gentamicin.
   E. chloramphenicol.

17. A 22 year old female developed a urinary tract infection during her honeymoon. Urine culture yielded a gram positive coccus inpairs and chains which grew of blood agar producing alpha hemolysis. Optochin did not inhibit growth. The isolated organism can be identified as

   A. *Staphylococcus aureus.*
   B. *Enterobacter aerogenes.*
   C. *Enterococcus faecalis.*
   D. *Streptococcus pyogenes.*

18. In aspergillosis, what is the most probable portal of entry?

   A. puncture wound
   B. Blood
   C. Lungs
   D. Gastrointestinal tract
   E. Insect bite

19. The addition of DNAse to a donor-recipient mixture will inhibit which of the following gene transfers?

   A. Transduction
   B. Transformation
   C. Transposition
   D. Conjugation

20. Specialized transduction

   A. transfers all genes of the chromosome with equal frequency.
   B. requires competent recipient cells.
   C. is accomplished with phage particles induction of lysogens.
   D. is always accomplished with virulent bacteriophages.
   E. requires cell to cell contact of donor and recipient.

21. The predominant virulence factor of *Shigella dysenteriae* is a (an)

   A. enterotoxin/cytotoxin.
   B. polysaccharide capsule.
   C. flagella.
   D. potent endotoxin.
   E. plasmid mediated antibiotic resistance factor.

22. *Staphylococcus aureus* would be the most likely cause of meningitis in which patient described below?

A. AIDS patient
B. Neonate
C. Alcoholic with history of recent head trauma
D. Child in kindergarten
E. Neurosurgical post-operative patient

23. The treatment of choice for disseminated candidiasis is

A. flucytosine.
B. potassium iodide.
C. miconazole.
D. nystatin.
E. metronidazole.

24. Immunodeficiency resulting in increased susceptibility to viral and fungal infections is due primarily to a deficiency in

A. macrophages.
B. B cells.
C. T cells.
D. neutrophils.
E. complement.

25. The major antiphagocytic cell wall component of *Streptococcus pyogenes* is

A. Hyaluronic acid
B. Peptidoglycan
C. M protein
D. DNAse
E. Erythrogenic toxin

26. Which of the following is a sporogenic obligate anaerobe?

A. *Bacillus anthracis*
B. *Bacteroides fragilis*
C. *Clostridium botulinum*
D. *Diphyllobothrium latum*
E. *Ehrlichia canis*

27. The infectious particle in chlamydial infections is a (an)

A. spore.
B. bacterial cell.
C. reticulate body.
D. elementary body.

28. In Gram negatives, lipopolysaccharide largely replaces phospholipid in the

A. inner membrane.
B. cell nucleus.
C. mesosomes.
D. outer membrane.
E. capsule.

29. One of the components of the bacterial cytoplasmic membrane is the

A. active transport system.
B. porin channel.
C. lipopolysaccharide.
D. peptidoglycan.
E. capsule.

30. Cell wall teichoic acids

A. occur in Gram negative bacteria only.
B. of *Streptococcus pyogenes* are involved in adherence to host cells.
C. are responsible for the rigidity of the cell wall.
D. act as molecular sieves.
E. are responsible for the endotoxin activity of lipopolysaccharide.

31. Phenol and its derivatives are excellent

A. for the elimination of spores
B. examples of quaternary ammonium detergents
C. vegetative cell poisons
D. topical antibiotics
E. food preservatives

32. Insertional inactivation as it applies to an in vitro recombinant DNA experiment refers to the

A. introduction of DNA into a restriction site within a specific gene, which results in inactivation of that gene.
B. inactivation of R factors by insertion sequences such that autonomous replication is inhibited.
C. introduction of mutations in DNA.
D. removal of intervening sequences from mRNA by RNA-splicing enzymes.

221

33. Damage to DNA, caused by bifunctional alkylating agents that damage both strands of DNA is repaired by

   A. photoeactivation.
   B. excision repair.
   C. direct repair.
   D. recombination.
   E. microinsertion.

34. Eukaryotic genes can be expressed in prokaryotes

   A. because the promotors are the same in both types of organisms.
   B. with the aid of prokaryotic promotors and ribosome binding sites.
   C. because prokaryotes are able to splice out the intervening sequences.
   D. because both have the same ribosomes.
   E. because DNA is DNA.

35. Administration of pooled human gamma globulin to prevent type A viral (infectious) hepatitis is an example of

   A. active, natural immunity
   B. active, artificial immunity
   C. passive, natural immunity
   D. passive, artificial immunity

36. A viral inhibitor that blocks myxovirus penetration into the cell is

   A. ribavirin.
   B. virazole.
   C. azidothymidine.
   D. IUDR.
   E. amantidine.

37. The large number of serotypes has prevented the use of a vaccine for which of the following viruses?

   A. Rhabdovirus
   B. Rubella
   C. Reo
   D. Rhino
   E. Polio

38. Hereditary angioneurotic edema is a disease caused by a deficiency of

   A. C3 proactivator
   B. C1 esterase inhibitor
   C. C1 esterase
   D. C3 convertase

39. Which of the following characteristics is associated with severe combined immune deficiency?

   A. Macrophages may be absent
   B. Gamma globulin levels will be normal
   C. Lymphocytes in germinal centers are depleted
   D. Abundant lymphocytes are seen in paracortical areas

40. Which of the following normal flora agents is etiologically associated with pseudomembranous enterocolitis?

   A. *Clostridium dificile*
   B. *Branhamella catarrhalis*
   C. *Corynebacterium diphtheriae*
   D. *Streptococcus mutans*

41. *Haemophilus influenzae*

   A. is a Gram positive rod.
   B. contains endotoxin (lipopolysaccharide).
   C. is a leading cause of croup.
   D. is uniformly susceptible to beta lactam antibiotics.
   E. grows well on nutrient agar plates.

42. Bacterial exotoxins are

   A. poor immunogens.
   B. cell wall surface components of Gram negative bacteria.
   C. easily detoxified.
   D. complexes of Lipid A and polysaccharide.
   E. cell wall surface components of Gram positive bacteria.

43. During a routine pelvic examination, a woman is found to have a tender, open lesion on the vagina. The patient states that she had similar lesions 12 mo. previously. The causative agent is most likely to be

   A. Echovirus.
   B. Coxsackievirus.
   C. Rubella virus.
   D. Herpes simplex virus.
   E. Measles virus.

44. Retroviruses are unique among all viruses in that

    A. the mature virus contains a strand of RNA and a strand of DNA.
    B. they can carry out replication of their genomes extracellularly within intact vesicles.
    C. they contain reverse transcriptase in the virion.
    D. they are nonantigenic.
    E. the mature virus contains no nucleic acid.

45. A 3-year-old child has a temperature of 38.3°C (101°F). On examination, discrete vesiculoulcerative lesions (Koplik's spots) are noted on the mucous membranes of the mouth. The most probable diagnosis is

    A. rubella.
    B. herpangina.
    C. measles.
    D. herpetic gingivostomatitis
    E. scarlet fever.

DIRECTIONS (ITEMS 46-55): Each of the numbered items or incomplete statements in this section is negatively phrased, as indicated by a capitalized word such as **NOT, LEAST**, or **EXCEPT**. Select the **ONE** lettered answer or completion that is **BEST** in each case.

---

46. All of the following concerning transformations are true **EXCEPT**

    A. native double stranded DNA is the most efficient form of transforming DNA.
    B. DNAse addition to the transformation mixture will result in no recombinants.
    C. a period of competence is generally necessary for recipients to take up the DNA.
    D. enzymes are required for the successful recombination occuring in transformation.
    E. DNA cannot enter F+ cells which contain pili.

47. Intereferon(s) do all of the following **EXCEPT**

    A. induce an antiviral state in cells.
    B. are produced by lymphoid cells.
    C. can be induced by animal cells exposed to inactive rotavirus.
    D. protect animals from prion attack.

48. Which of the following vaccine/recipient pairs would be the **LEAST** appropriate?

    A. Hepatitis B vaccine/Dentists.
    B. Measles vaccine/Pre-school children.
    C. Influenza vaccine/Nursing home residents.
    D. Rubella vaccine/Prostitute

49. Virulence factors of *Pseudomonas aeruginosa* include all of the following **EXCEPT**

    A. a potent exotoxin that inhibits protein synthesis.
    B. elastase, which plays a role in dissolving surfactant.
    C. an antiphagocytic slime layer.
    D. lipopolysaccharide endotoxin.
    E. a potent exotoxin that activates adenyl cyclase.

50. Which of the following is **not true** for carcinoembryonic antigen (CEA)?

    A. It is elevated in some heavy smokers
    B. An elevated CEA in a patient with carcinoma of the colon is a poor prognostic sign
    C. An elevated CEA level establishes the diagnosis of carcinoma of the colon
    D. CEA levels may be used to monitor the effectiveness of therapy

51. A 6-year-old farm boy develops restlessness, hallucinations, and convulsions and dies 2 days later. At autopsy the only significant finding is eosinophilic inclusions in neurons. These findings are consistent with all of the following **EXCEPT**

    A. rabies.
    B. varicella infection of the CNS.
    C. herpes simplex encephalitis.
    D. coxsackie virus encephalitis.

52. Orthomyxoviruses are correctly described by all of the following statments **EXCEPT**

    A. being of three antigenic types (A, B, and C).
    B. having a segmented genome.
    C. typed according to the ribonucleo-protein in the virion.
    D. having RNA as their genetic information.
    E. one member of the family causes mumps.

53. Extracellular products of *Streptococcus* spp. include all of the following **EXCEPT**

    A. DNAse.
    B. glucosyl transferase.
    C. hyaluronic acid.
    D. hyaluronidase.
    E. enterotoxin.

54. The aminoglycoside antibiotics do all of the following **EXCEPT**

    A. prevent initiation of protein synthesis.
    B. are inactivated by phosphorylation in resistant bacteria.
    C. cause damage to the eight cranial nerve.
    D. react with the 80S ribosome.
    E. are inactivated by adenylation.

55. Replication of HIV would be blocked by all of the following **EXCEPT**

    A. Inhibitors of RNA-dependent DNA polymerases
    B. Inhibitors of DNA-dependent RNA polymerases
    C. Azidothymidine
    D. Inhibitors of DNA-dependent DNA polymerase

DIRECTIONS (Items 56-84): Each set of matching questions in this section consists of a list of up to 26 lettered options, followed by several numbered items. For each numbered item, select the ONE lettered option that is most closely associated with it. **EACH LETTERED OPTION MAY BE SELECTED ONCE, MORE THAN ONCE, OR NOT AT ALL.**

MATCH THE PATIENT WITH THE VACCINE.

    A. Toxoid
    B. Live, attenuated organism
    C. Killed, attenuated organism
    D. Killed, virulent organism
    E. Purified capsular carbohydrate
    F. Pilus

    G. Recombinant DNA product
    H. Purified outer membrane protein
    I. Purified protein derivative
    J. Membrane siderophores
    K. Envelop hemagglutinins
    L. Human gamma globulin

56. A Wyoming cattleman receives a serious wound when he is bucked into a wire fence. He refuses medical treatment and develops *rhisus sardonicus* 3 weeks later. This could have been prevented if he had received what vaccine?

57. A newly inducted army recriut reports to Fort Sill for processing. He will receive what vaccine to protect him from epidemic meningitis?

58. A nine day old infant is brought to the missionary hospital in Zaire. The child has an obviously infected umbilical stump and is experiencing severe opisthotonus. This could have been prevented if the mother had received what type of vaccine?

A. Inhibits transpeptidation

B. Inhibits peptidyl transferase

C. Blocks initiation of protein synthesis

D. Inhibits DNA-dependent RNA polymerase

E. Blocks binding of aminoacyl tRNA

F. Inhibits DNA gyrase

G. Inhibits dihydrofolate reductase

H. Blocks mycolic acid synthesis

I. Inhibits dihydrofolate synthetase

J. Blocks chitin synthesis

K. Intercalates into cell membrane

L. Blocks ergosterol synthesis

59. Cephalosporins

60. Aminoglycosides

61. Fluoroquinolones

62. Trimethoprim

A. Bruton's agammaglobulinemia

B. Systemic lupus erythematosus

C. Grave's disease

D. Insulin dependent diabetes mellitus

E. CREST syndrome

F. Sjogren's syndrome

G. Serum sickness

H. Asthma

I. Idiopathic thrombocytopenia purpura

J. Juvenile rheumatoid arthritis

K. Hashimoto's thyroiditis

L. Chronic granulomatous disease

M. Multiple sclerosis

N. Acquired immune deficiency syndrome

63. A 24-year-old ski instructor has a 3-week history of joint pain that has hampered her work. She has recently developed a rash over the malar aspect of her face. Her serum contains high levels of antibodies to dsDNA.

64. A 36-year-old highly nervous housewife presents with exophthalmus. The pertinent laboratory findings are those suggestive of hyperthyroidism.

65. A 42-year old school teacher presents with a complaint of dryness of the eyes, mouth, nose, and vagina. She has a twelve year history of arthritic problems. Serum studies reveal the presence of antinuclear antibodies, rheumatoid factor, and autoantibodies against salivary duct antigens.

66. A 46-year-old accountant presents with a unique complex of symptoms; calcinosis, Raynaud's phenomenon, esophageal dysmotility, sclerodactyly, and telangiectasia. Anti-centromere autoantibodies are present in the serum.

FOR EACH PATIENT DESCRIBED BELOW, SELECT THE MOST APPROPRIATE THERAPEUTIC AGENT.

A.	Trimethoprim/sulfamethoxazole	I.	Iodo-deoxyuridine
B.	Ribavirin	J.	Oxacillin
C.	Chloramphenicol	K.	Ketoconazole
D.	Dexamethasone	L.	Lincomycin
E.	Potassium iodide	M.	Penicillin
F.	Acyclovir	O.	Amantadine
G.	Isoniazid/rifampin	P.	Metronidazole
H.	Interferon		

67. Twenty six year-old Sioux Indian who has lived on the Pine Ridge reservation all his life has developed night sweats and a low grade fever. He has shortness of breath and a cough which is productive of rusty sputum (hemoptosis). Acid fast bacilli are seen on stain of the sputum.

68. Eighteen year-old football player has recently been ill with flu-like disease. He now complains of shortness of breath and a fever of 39.4C. Gram stain of the sputum reveals Gram positive cocci in random clusters.

69. This 3 month-old girl was born prematurely at a gestational age of 31 weeks. She has been hospitalized all her life. She recently has developed signs of bronchitis which have progressed to severe interstitial pneumonitis. Immunofluorescent examination of exfloiated cells in respiratory tract secretions reveals numerous syncytial masses with intracytoplasmic inclusion bodies.

70. A 59-year-old botanist was "pricked" while tending to his rose garden. Two weeks later he developed a draining sore on his hand. The lesion spread up the lymphatics to involve other nodes in the forearm.

71. A 37 year-old bartender presents with a painful vesicular eruption that has a dermatomal distribution. As the patient is currently taking corticosteroidal drugs to control a severe asthmatic attack, vigorous therapy is undertaken to prevent the development of systemic disease.

72. A 29 year-old exotic dancer complains of vaginal itching and burning. A foul smelling greenish fluid is collected from her vagina and submitted to the Microbiology laboratory for culture and sensitivity studies.

73. The patient is a 24 year-old woman with lower abdominal pain of 3 days duration. The symptoms have intensified during the last 24 hours and she now is feverish and her pain, which is severe, is localized to her left-lower-quadrant; adnexal tenderness is noted and a purulent discharge is sampled from the cervical os. Gram stain reveals numerous PMNs and Gram negative rods. The organisms are reported out as "Obligate Anaerobes" by the Microbiology lab.

74. This 14 year-old young man has severely inflamed tonsil's and pharynx. A culture yields gram positive cocci in chains of 6-8. The organism is inhibited by bacitracin.

226

A.	Alpha interferon	G.	Interleukin 4
B.	Beta interferon	H.	Interleukin 6
C.	Gamma interferon	I.	Interleukin 8
D.	Tumor necrosis factor α	J.	Interleukin 10
E.	Interleukin 1	K.	Tumor necrosis factor β
F.	Interleukin 2	L.	Perforin

75. Increases expression of MHC antigens on cells of the body

76. Lymphotoxin

77. Immune interferon

78. Inhibits cytokine synthesis by Th 1 cells

79. Chemotactic monokine

80. Down regulates Th 2 cells

81. Increases Fc receptors on macrophages

82. Major role in class switching

83. Endogenous pyrogen

84. Polymerizes into membrane on target cells

A.	Hepatitis A virus	F.	Molluscum contagiosum
B.	Hepatitis B virus	G.	Papilloma virus
C.	Hepatitis C virus	H.	Parvovirus
D.	Hepatitis D virus	I.	Epstien Barr virus
E.	Hepatitis E virus	J.	Human Immunodeficiency virus

85. Kaposi's sarcoma

86. Nasopharyngeal carcinoma

87. Burkitt's lymphoma

88. Cervical carcinoma

A.	IgE	E.	IgD
B.	IgA	F.	sIgA
C.	IgG	G.	IgM (7s)
D.	IgM (19s)	H.	dimeric IgA

89. Has a half life of approximately 21 days

90. Predominant antibody in colostrum

91. Crosses the placenta in humans

A.	Picornaviruses	F.	Retroviruses
B.	Orthomyxoviruses	G.	Poxviruses
C.	Rotaviruses	H.	Adenoviruses
D.	Hepadnaviruses	I.	Herpesviruses
E.	Rhabdoviruses	J.	Parvoviruses

92. Virions that contain double-stranded RNA that is in several pieces.

93. Virions carry single-stranded RNA that is in several pieces and is complementary to mRNA (is antimessenger).

94. Purified, naked viral nucleic acid is infectious if inserted into cells.

95. Virions contain a partially double-stranded circular DNA.

A.	*Aspergillus fumigatus*	F.	*Penicillium notatum*
B.	*Pseudomonas aeruginosa*	G.	*Cryptococcus neoformans*
C.	*Staphylococcus aureus*	H.	*Toxoplasma gondii*
D.	*Propionibacterium acnes*	I.	*Pasteurella multocida*
E.	*Streptococcus pneumoniae*	J.	*Mycobacterium tuberculosis*

96.   A 37-year-old farmer who is currently on immunotherapy for acute lymphocytic leukemia has developed pneumonitis with hemoptosis. He reports that he has been smoking "grass" to control the nausea associated with his therapy. On X-ray a lesion is seen which is described by the radiologist as a "fungus ball". The agent most likely is

97.   A Fireman was severely injured after being trapped by the collapse of a burning barn. He was sent to the Burn Unit of a metropolitan hospital for care. Nine days after admission he developed a severe infection of the dorsal surface of his right arm where he had received severe third degree burns. Tfhe most likely agent to be isolated from the exudate is

98.   A 43 year old Mexican businessman has recently moved to the United States to work in the World Bank. On routine physical examination for insurance a spot is noted on his lung in the upper right lobe. He reports that he has recently been experiencing night sweats and has lost 18 pounds in the past 6 months. There is a 16 mm area of induration around the site of a ppd skin test (read at 72 hours).

99.   This 27 year old mother of three pre-schoolers presents with an ugly lesion on her right wrist. It is "angry" and filled with pus. There appears to be a central core which she reports is the site of a bite she received from a neighbor's cat while attempting to remove the animal from her babies' play house.

100.   A 23 year old accountant suffered a splenic rupture in an auto accident which occurred while he was returning from his Doctor's office where a diagnosis of infectious mononucleosis was made. Splenectomy was performed due to the extensive damage to the organ. Four months later he develops a high fever with hypotension and is hospitalized with a tentative diagnosis of septicemia.

KEY

1.	A	16.	B	31.	C	46.	E	61.	F	76.	C	91.	C
2.	B	17.	C	32.	A	47.	D	62.	G	77.	G	92.	C
3.	D	18.	C	33.	D	48.	D	63.	B	78.	E	93.	B
4.	A	19.	B	34.	B	49.	E	64.	C	79.	L	94.	A
5.	C	20.	C	35.	D	50.	D	65.	F	80.	K	95.	D
6.	B	21.	A	36.	E	51.	D	66.	E	81.	C	96.	A
7.	B	22.	E	37.	D	52.	E	67.	G	82.	J	97	B
8.	A	23.	A	38.	B	53.	E	68.	J	83.	I	98	J
9.	B	24.	C	39.	D	54.	D	69.	B	84.	C	99.	I
10.	B	25.	C	40.	A	55.	D	70.	E	85.	J	100.	E
11.	B	26.	C	41.	B	56.	A	71.	F	86.	I		
12.	E	27.	D	42.	C	57.	E	72.	P	87.	I		
13.	A	28.	D	43.	D	58.	A	73.	P	88.	G		
14.	A	29.	A	44.	C	59.	A	74.	M	89.	C		
15.	D	30.	B	45.	C	60.	C	75.	C	90.	B		